Neurosurgery Primary Board Review

Ross C. Puffer, MD
Neurosurgical Resident
Department of Neurosurgery
Mayo Clinic
Rochester, Minnesota, USA

217 illustrations

Thieme
Stuttgart • New York • Delhi • Rio de Janeiro

Executive Editor: Timothy Hiscock
Managing Editor: Sapna Rastogi
Director, Editorial Services: Mary Jo Casey
Production Editor: Shivika
International Production Director: Andreas
    Schabert
International Marketing Director: Fiona Henderson
Editorial Director: Sue Hodgson
International Sales Director: Louisa Turrell
Director of Sales, North America: Mike Roseman
Senior Vice President and Chief Operating Officer:
    Sarah Vanderbilt
President: Brian D. Scanlan

Library of Congress Cataloging-in-Publication Data

© 2019 Thieme Medical Publishers, Inc. Thieme
Publishers New York
333 Seventh Avenue, New York, NY 10001 USA
+1 800 782 3488, customerservice@thieme.com

Thieme Publishers Stuttgart
Rüdigerstrasse 14, 70469 Stuttgart, Germany
+49 [0]711 8931 421, customerservice@thieme.de

Thieme Publishers Delhi
A-12, Second Floor, Sector-2, Noida-201301
Uttar Pradesh, India
+91 120 45 566 00, customerservice@thieme.in

Thieme Publishers Rio, Thieme Publicações Ltda.
Edifício Rodolpho de Paoli, 25º andar
Av. Nilo Peçanha, 50 – Sala 2508
Rio de Janeiro 20020-906, Brasil
+55 21 3172 2297

Cover design: Thieme Publishing Group
Typesetting by DiTech Process Solutions Pvt. Ltd., India

Printed in USA by King Printing Company, Inc.
5 4 3 2 1

ISBN 978-1-62623-927-2

Also available as an e-book:
eISBN 978-1-62623-928-9

Important note: Medicine is an ever-changing science undergoing continual development. Research and clinical experience are continually expanding our knowledge, in particular our knowledge of proper treatment and drug therapy. Insofar as this book mentions any dosage or application, readers may rest assured that the authors, editors, and publishers have made every effort to ensure that such references are in accordance with **the state of knowledge at the time of production of the book.**

Nevertheless, this does not involve, imply, or express any guarantee or responsibility on the part of the publishers in respect to any dosage instructions and forms of applications stated in the book. **Every user is requested to examine carefully** the manufacturers' leaflets accompanying each drug and to check, if necessary in consultation with a physician or specialist, whether the dosage schedules mentioned therein or the contraindications stated by the manufacturers differ from the statements made in the present book. Such examination is particularly important with drugs that are either rarely used or have been newly released on the market. Every dosage schedule or every form of application used is entirely at the user's own risk and responsibility. The authors and publishers request every user to report to the publishers any discrepancies or inaccuracies noticed. If errors in this work are found after publication, errata will be posted at www.thieme.com on the product description page.

Some of the product names, patents, and registered designs referred to in this book are in fact registered trademarks or proprietary names even though specific reference to this fact is not always made in the text. Therefore, the appearance of a name without designation as proprietary is not to be construed as a representation by the publisher that it is in the public domain.

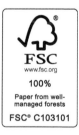

This book is dedicated to my wife, Emily, for her unwavering support through all the years of my training. To my fellow neurosurgery residents; remember they can always make it a little harder, but they cannot stop the clock.

Contents

Foreword

It is an honor for me to christen this book by Dr. Ross Puffer for the ABNS written (primary) examination. For nearly two decades, I have been an enthusiastic teacher for multiple written and oral neurosurgical board preparation courses in neurosurgery. This book is the end product of a casual comment to Ross approximately 1 year ago—that there was a void for a contemporary neurosurgical review book addressing the seven sections of the exam (neuroanatomy, neurosciences, neuropathology, neuroimaging, clinical neurology, neurosurgery, critical care/fundamental clinical skills), and core competencies. Both the comprehensive nature and the quick turnaround time of this book are testaments to Dr. Puffer's innate talents.

I have known and admired Ross for 10 years: first as a medical school student and more recently as a neurosurgical resident at the Mayo Clinic, an institution where his parents have been on staff—his father, a family physician, and his mother, a radiologist. Ross has been an exemplary student and resident, demonstrating his ability to absorb, process, and apply a large amount of information with ease. He has consistently scored in the 99th percentile on standardized examinations (including the targeted ABNS primary examination). His clinical performance demonstrates his evidence-based approach to patients and compassionate care. His knowledge of the literature combined with his organizational skills have helped him become a prolific researcher, answering clinically relevant questions during his abundant "free time." Equally as impressive has been his ability to educate and mentor, and serve as a role model. He knows how to simplify complex concepts into smaller morsels that can be digested.

In short, this Q & A review book and question bank will be a great resource not only for residents preparing for this important primary examination, but also for learners at all levels throughout their careers as practicing neurosurgeons.

Robert J. Spinner, MD

Preface

Those who train in medicine these days understand that to complete training (medical school, residency, and fellowship), one must become a professional test taker. At every level, there are one or more standardized tests that act as gateways to residency programs, training, and board certification. On occasion, trainees joke that if only patients could present as a multiple choice question, the practice of medicine would be much easier. My personal experience navigating these tests has involved completing practice questions before each test, sometimes thousands of practice questions. Practice questions allow the student to closely simulate the examination experience, and often serve as a powerful identifier of areas in need of further study.

This book was created from a set of questions I wrote while studying for the American Board of Neurological Surgery (ABNS) primary written examination in 2017. Some questions are available currently to students, but residents can benefit from a larger bank of practice questions to study from. The field is rapidly advancing, and the material and format of the ABNS primary examination is changing constantly. Exam preparation materials should evolve along with the test and the field of neurosurgery in general. Many references and texts are now accessible online, and on the go. While this question book is in print, the entirety of the question bank will also be available online

with simulated test software, to allow the learner to closely mimic the test experience, as well as take advantage of direct reference links and high-quality images. The question bank consists of 1,575 questions, 1,200 of which are designed for general study, as well as a stand-alone, 375-question practice examination with 120 images taken from the Thieme image library. The practice examination contains the exact number of questions as the current examination, and they are categorized into the same subjects as listed on the ABNS primary examination website. The main question bank contains 1,200 questions, 264 images from the Thieme image library, and is divided into the same subjects as the primary examination itself.

My hope is that making these questions available to residents studying for the ABNS primary examination will help improve the number of available practice questions, as well as provide a set of questions relevant to the current examination. The online version of these questions should be welcomed by residents who are used to standardized examination preparation via online question banks, as is standard for these tests in medical school. I would like to thank Thieme for their help in the production of this text as well as the production of an online test taking software system that will allow residents to simulate the examination environment better than I was able to with currently available resources.

Ross C. Puffer, MD

I Questions

1 Neurosurgery

1.

You are evaluating an 82-year-old man who takes 325 mg of aspirin daily for coronary artery disease. He presented to the emergency department with a headache and sleepiness. CT is shown below. What is the most likely diagnosis?

Use the following figure to answer questions 1 through 5:

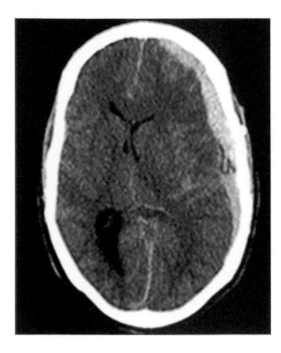

A. Epidural hematoma
B. Subdural hematoma
C. Intraparenchymal hematoma
D. Traumatic subarachnoid hemorrhage

2.

You are evaluating an 82-year-old man who takes 325 mg of aspirin daily for coronary artery disease. He presented to the emergency department with a headache and sleepiness. Refer to CT shown in Question 1. How long has this bleed likely been present?

A. 1 to 3 days
B. 4 days to 2 weeks
C. 2 weeks to 3 months
D. > 3 months

3.

You are evaluating an 82-year-old man with a history of a mechanical aortic valve. He presented to the emergency department with a headache and sleepiness. His GCS is 13 (E3, V4, M6). Refer to CT shown in Question 1. What is the next best step?

A. Intubate
B. Bedside burr hole evacuation
C. Start levetiracetam
D. Check INR

4.

You are evaluating an 82-year-old man with a history of a mechanical aortic valve. He presented to the emergency department with a headache and sleepiness. His GCS is 13 (E3, V4, M6). Refer to CT shown in Question 1. You decide to intervene. What procedure would you recommend?

A. EVD insertion
B. Burr hole evacuation
C. Decompressive hemicraniotomy/ectomy
D. Posterior fossa decompression

5.

You are evaluating an 82-year-old man with a history of a mechanical aortic valve. He presented to the emergency department with a headache but is otherwise neurologically intact with a GCS of 15. What would you recommend?

A. EVD insertion
B. Admission/observation
C. Decompressive hemicraniotomy/ectomy
D. Discharge home from ED with 1 month follow-up head CT

6.

You see a 40-year-old man who was out drinking with friends and was involved in a car accident as an unrestrained passenger. He is sleepy in the trauma bay and his head CT is demonstrated below. What is the most likely diagnosis?

Use the following figure to answer questions 6 to 8 and 10:

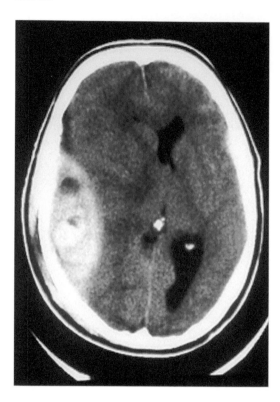

A. Chronic subdural hematoma
B. Acute subdural hematoma
C. Epidural hematoma
D. Traumatic subarachnoid hemorrhage

7.

You see a 40-year-old man who was out drinking with friends and was involved in a car accident as an unrestrained passenger. He is sleepy in the trauma bay and his head CT is demonstrated in Question 6. The injured vessel in this setting enters the skull through what foramen?

A. Foramen ovale
B. Foramen rotundum
C. Foramen spinosum
D. Foramen lacerum

8.

You see a 40-year-old man who was out drinking with friends and was involved in a car accident as an unrestrained passenger. He is sleepy in the trauma bay and his head CT is demonstrated in Question 6. What is the next best step?

A. EVD placement
B. Observation
C. Operative evacuation
D. Bedside burr hole drainage

9.

You see a 40-year-old man who was involved in a car accident as an unrestrained passenger. He is awake and responsive in the trauma bay (GCS 15) and his head CT is demonstrated below. What is the next best step?

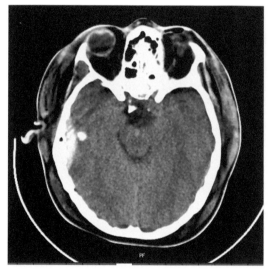

A. EVD placement
B. Observation/rescan
C. Operative evacuation
D. Bedside burr hole drainage

10.

You see a 40-year-old man who was involved in a car accident as an unrestrained passenger. He initially lost consciousness but EMTs reported that he woke up and was talking to them through transport. When you see him in the trauma bay he is no longer responding verbally and opens his eyes only to deep central stimulation. His head CT is demonstrated in Question 6. What is the next best step?

A. EVD placement
B. Observation/rescan
C. Operative evacuation
D. Intubate

11.

You are evaluating a 55-year-old woman who was involved in a car accident where she hit her head and she thinks she lost consciousness. On CT scan you see small hyperdensities in both frontal lobes concerning for small intraparenchymal hemorrhages. She has a GCS of 15. What should you recommend in your consult note?

A. Discharge home
B. Rescan in 6 hours
C. Rescan now
D. Start levetiracetam

12.

You are evaluating an 82-year-old man who takes 325 mg of aspirin daily for coronary artery disease. He presented to the emergency department with a headache and sleepiness. MRI is shown below. How long has this bleed likely been present?

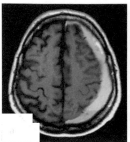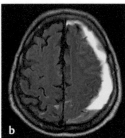

A. 1 day
B. 3 days
C. 1 week
D. > 3 weeks

13.

You are evaluating an 82-year-old man who takes 325 mg of aspirin daily for coronary artery disease. He presented to the emergency department with a headache and sleepiness. CT is shown below. What procedure would you recommend?

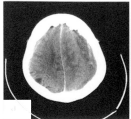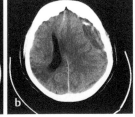

A. EVD placement
B. Burr hole evacuation
C. Decompressive hemicraniotomy/ectomy
D. Posterior fossa decompression

14.

You are seeing a 78-year-old man in your office who underwent drainage of a large, right-sided chronic subdural hematoma approximately 40 days ago. He has evidence of a residual subdural fluid collection. Approximately how many patients will still have a fluid collection after subdural drainage at 40 days?

A. 3%
B. 15%
C. 35%
D. 60%
E. 90%

15.

When evaluating patients with gunshot wounds to the head, bullet trajectory is important for prognostication. What trajectory has been found to be uniformly fatal in the civilian population?

A. Bifrontal trajectory
B. Holohemispheric trajectory
C. Biventricular trajectory
D. Transverse cerebellar trajectory

16.

You are asked to evaluate a 65-year-old patient who was discharged from the hospital 1 week ago after undergoing decompression of a right-sided subdural hematoma. She has noticed some clear drainage from her incision and has had a persistent, severe headache all day. Head CT is demonstrated below. What is the diagnosis?

Use the following figure to answer questions 16 and 17:

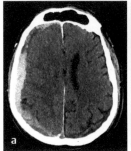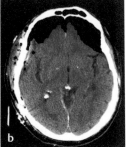

A. Subdural hematoma
B. Epidural hematoma
C. Tension pneumocephalus
D. Subdural empyema

17.

You are asked to evaluate a 65-year-old patient who was discharged from the hospital 1 week ago after undergoing decompression of a right-sided subdural hematoma. She has noticed some clear drainage from her incision and has had a persistent, severe headache all day. She prefers to keep her eyes closed and responds with one-word answers only. Head CT is demonstrated in Question 16. What is the next best step?

A. Decompression
B. Lumbar drain
C. Discharge home
D. 100% FiO2 via nonrebreather

18.

You have been asked to act as the sideline physician for a local high school football game. One of the players takes a big hit and appears to initially walk to the wrong sideline. When you evaluate him he says that he doesn't remember the previous play. Should he be allowed to go back into the game?

A. Yes
B. No

19.

What is the normal range of intracranial pressure in adults (mm Hg)?

A. 1 to 4
B. 5 to 9
C. 10 to 15
D. 16 to 20

20.

How is cerebral perfusion pressure calculated?

A. $CPP = CMRO_2 + ICP$
B. $CPP = SBP - ICP$
C. $CPP = MAP - ICP$
D. $CPP = CBF - ICP$

21.

A 33-year-old man is attempting to perform BMX tricks on a bicycle and is not wearing a helmet. He goes over the handlebars and hits his head on a concrete surface. He loses consciousness at the scene but regains consciousness in the trauma bay and is GCS 15. CT is shown below. What is the next best step?

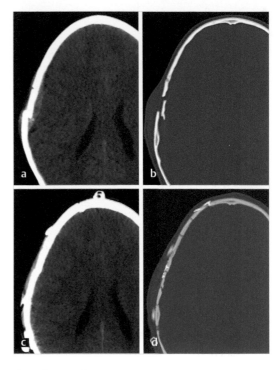

A. Observation
B. IV antibiotics
C. Operative elevation/debridement
D. Discharge home

22.

What is the most common type of temporal bone fracture?

A. Longitudinal
B. Transverse
C. Anterior
D. Lateral

23.

What type of temporal bone fracture is associated with VII nerve injury?

A. Longitudinal
B. Transverse
C. Anterior
D. Lateral

24.
You are seeing a patient in the trauma bay who was involved in a motor vehicle accident leading to a skull base fracture that appears to be a transverse temporal bone fracture. There is blood coming from the EAC and significant bruising around the ear/mastoid tip. On exam the patient is GCS 15, but has House-Brackmann grade VI left facial nerve function. What is the next best step?

A. Immediate surgical decompression
B. IV antibiotics
C. Start steroids
D. Repeat head CT

25.
You are seeing a patient in the trauma bay who was involved in a motor vehicle accident leading to a skull base fracture that appears to be a transverse fracture of the clivus. All of the following should be performed except?

A. CBC/Electrolyte panel
B. NG tube insertion
C. CT angiogram head and neck
D. Cervical spine CT

26.
What type of Lefort facial fracture has a high incidence of associated brain injury?

A. Type I
B. Type II
C. Type III
D. Type IV

27.
You are asked to see a 6-month-old infant who sustained a skull fracture after his older brother accidentally pulled down the flat screen TV that landed on the infant's head. CT scan is demonstrated below. The child is neurologically intact with no focal deficits. How would you manage this fracture?

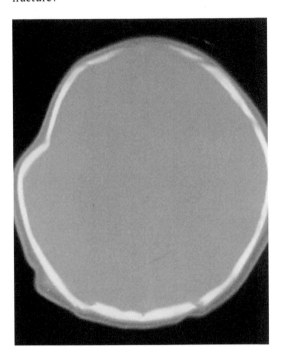

A. Operative elevation
B. Observation

28.
You are asked to see a 6-month-old infant who sustained a skull fracture after his older brother accidentally pulled down the flat screen TV that landed on the infant's head. Follow-up CT scan is demonstrated below. What is the diagnosis?

Use the following figure to answer questions 28 and 29:

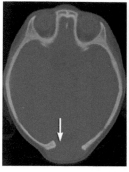 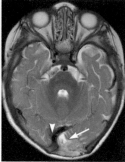

A. Growing skull fracture
B. Arachnoid cyst
C. Intraparenchymal hemorrhage
D. Normal bone healing

29.
You are asked to see a 6-month-old infant who sustained a skull fracture after his older brother accidentally pulled down the flat screen TV that landed on the infant's head. Follow-up CT scan is demonstrated in Question 28. What is the next best step?

A. Observation
B. Percutaneous drainage
C. Cranioplasty
D. Circumferential craniotomy and dural repair

30.
You are asked to see a 6-month-old infant who is being worked up for suspected non-accidental trauma. What is the most common intracranial manifestation of non-accidental trauma?

A. Diffuse axonal injury
B. Bilateral subdural hematomas
C. Intraparenchymal hemorrhage
D. Epidural hematoma

31.
What is the most common reason for retinal hemorrhages on fundoscopy in an infant?

A. Nonaccidental trauma
B. Benign subdural effusion in infants
C. Acute high altitude sickness
D. Acute ICP increase

32.
You are seeing a 25-year-old man who was involved in a car accident where he hit his head on the windshield and lost consciousness. What marker has been shown to be associated with acute traumatic brain injury?

A. PTEN
B. GFAP
C. Amyloid precursor protein
D. Tau protein

33.
You have been following a 55-year-old man with severe traumatic brain injury and depressed GCS for the last 48 hours. A bolt was placed, and over the last 6 hours ICP has been elevated to 30 despite aggressive medical management. According to the DECRA trial, what is the best next step?

A. Continued medical management
B. Withdrawal of care
C. Decompressive hemicraniectomy
D. Posterior fossa decompression

34.
You are performing a decompressive hemicraniectomy for a patient with evidence of impending herniation. What is the most important aspect of the craniectomy to decrease the risk of uncal herniation?

A. AP diameter > 12 cm
B. Drilling to the edge of the sagittal sinus
C. Drilling to the floor of the middle fossa
D. Intraoperative EVD placement

35.
Which of these options is not a part of Cushing's triad (signs of acute increased intracranial pressure)?

A. Hypotension
B. Hypertension
C. Bradycardia
D. Irregular respirations

36.
You are seeing a patient in the trauma bay with evidence of acute increased ICP who has subsequently been intubated. You are taking the patient to the OR for decompression. In order to temporize the situation, you sit up the patient's head of bed and tell the anesthesiologist to hyperventilate in order to decrease intracranial pressure. How long will this technique work?

A. ~ 1 minute
B. ~ 30 minutes
C. ~ 12 hours
D. ~ 24 hours
E. ~ 48 hours

37.
You are seeing a patient in the trauma bay with evidence of acute increased ICP who has subsequently been intubated. You are taking the patient to the OR for decompression. In order to temporize the situation, you sit up the patient's head of bed and tell the anesthesiologist to hyperventilate in order to decrease intracranial pressure. What is the target PaCO$_2$ you are aiming for?

A. 16 to 20 mm Hg
B. 21 to 25 mm Hg
C. 26 to 30 mm Hg
D. 31 to 35 mm Hg
E. 36 to 40 mm Hg

38.
You are medically managing a patient with persistent increased intracranial pressure using scheduled mannitol, 0.5 g/kg Q6H. You are appropriately checking serum osmolality during this treatment. What serum osmolality measurement would make you stop giving mannitol?

A. 306
B. 312
C. 318
D. 324

39.
You have been emergently consulted by neurology in a patient with a subarachnoid hemorrhage who has evidence of acute hydrocephalus and you feel that an EVD is warranted. What is a good approximation of where you should perform your bedside burr hole?

A. 8 cm back from the nasion, mid-pupillary line
B. 11 cm back from the nasion, mid-pupillary line
C. 14 cm back from the nasion, mid-pupillary line
D. 3 cm up from the pinna, 3 cm posterior

40.
You are taking care of a patient with persistently elevated intracranial pressure despite mannitol administration. You decide to utilize hypertonic saline, but the patient currently only has a peripheral IV. What is the highest concentration of hypertonic saline you can safely give through a peripheral IV?

A. 1.5%
B. 3%
C. 7%
D. 23.4%

41.
What is the approximate volume of CSF within the ventricular system at any given time?

A. 100 mL
B. 150 mL
C. 200 mL
D. 250 mL

42.
You see a patient in the trauma bay that opens his eyes to painful stimulation, localizes to that painful stimulation, and mutters incomprehensible words. What is the GCS?

A. 8
B. 10
C. 12
D. 14
E. 15

43.
You see a patient in the trauma bay that was intubated during transport for airway concerns, does not open his eyes to painful stimulation, and externally rotates/extends both upper extremities during that painful stimulation. What is the GCS?

A. 4t
B. 6t
C. 8t
D. 3t
E. 14t

44.
You are managing the care of a patient who has elevated ICP, hydrocephalus, and has had an EVD placed. Your staff wants you to move the EVD to 10 mm Hg, but the EVD catheter only has markings for cm H$_2$O. What should you set the EVD height to?

A. 8.7 cm H$_2$O
B. 17.4 cm H$_2$O
C. 13.6 cm H$_2$O
D. 21.4 cm H$_2$O

45.

What type of ICP waves are associated with elevations of ICP > 50 mm Hg for 5 to 20 minutes accompanied by elevations in mean arterial pressure?

A. Lundberg A waves
B. Lundberg B waves
C. Lundberg C waves
D. Lundberg D waves
E. Lundberg E waves

46.

Which peak of the ICP waveform gives you information about the compliance of the ventricular system?

A. P1
B. P2
C. P3
D. P4
E. P5

47.

In patients with elevated ICP, what should be the goal cerebral perfusion pressure?

A. > 20
B. > 50
C. > 100
D. > 150
E. > 200

48.

In a patient with elevated ICP (25 mm Hg) in the setting of severe traumatic brain injury, what should be the goal mean arterial pressure?

A. 45
B. 85
C. 115
D. 145
E. 165

49.

You are asked to evaluate a patient in the trauma bay that is unresponsive. He is intubated, does not open his eyes, and exhibits no movement of the upper or lower extremities even to deep painful stimulation of the nail bed. What is the GCS?

A. 0
B. 3
C. 6
D. 9
E. 12

50.

What medical therapy is thought to provide the maximum drop in $CMRO_2$ and CBF in patients with severely increased ICP in the setting of trauma?

A. Mannitol
B. Hypertonic saline
C. Propofol
D. Pentobarbital
E. Ketamine

51.

You are evaluating a 33-year-old man who experienced a first-time seizure; subsequent MRI was performed and is demonstrated below. If you decided to operate on this patient, what operative adjunct would be useful in this case?

Use the following figure to answer questions 51 and 52:

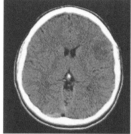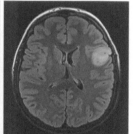
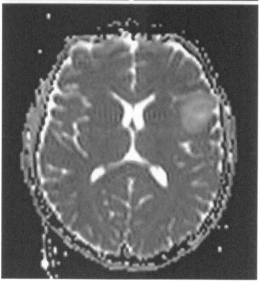

A. Motor mapping
B. Diffusion tensor imaging
C. Awake language mapping
D. Somatosensory evoked potentials
E. EMG

52.
You are evaluating a 33-year-old man who experienced a first-time seizure; subsequent MRI was performed and is demonstrated in Question 51. What further imaging study might be helpful in this case?

A. PET scan
B. Diffusion tensor imaging
C. Functional MRI
D. Perfusion MRI
E. Perfusion C

53.
You are evaluating a 45-year-old man who experienced a first-time seizure; subsequent MRI was performed and is demonstrated below. What would be useful during surgical resection of this mass?

Use the following figure to answer question 53:

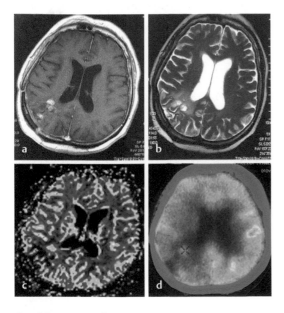

A. Motor mapping
B. Awake language mapping
C. Somatosensory evoked potentials
D. EMG

54.
You are operating on a 55-year-old man with a low-grade astrocytoma of the posterior frontal lobe and you are utilizing motor mapping to identify the motor structures. What monitoring finding alerts you to the location of the motor strip?

A. Doubling of signal amplitude
B. Signal dampening
C. Phase reversal
D. Phase doubling

55.
You are operating on a 55-year-old man with a low-grade astrocytoma of the posterior frontal lobe and you are utilizing motor mapping to identify the motor structures. Intraoperative recordings are demonstrated below. What electrode is located on the motor strip in this image?

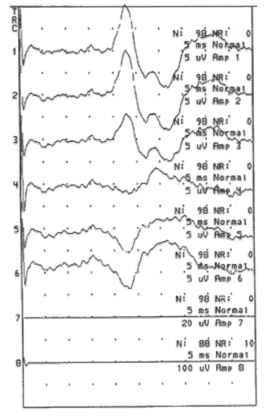

A. 2
B. 3
C. 4
D. 5
E. 6

56.
What is the most common tumor of the central nervous system?

A. Meningioma
B. Metastases
C. Glioblastoma
D. Lymphoma
E. Low-grade glioma

57.
What is the most common metastatic tumor to the brain?

A. Lymphoma
B. Lung
C. Colorectal
D. Melanoma
E. Renal

58.
What is the most common metastatic tumor to the brain in females?

A. Melanoma
B. Lung
C. Colorectal
D. Breast
E. Renal

59.
A 66-year-old woman presents to your clinic with a first-time seizure and an MRI was performed which is demonstrated below. What is the next best step?

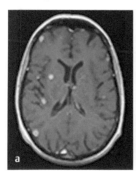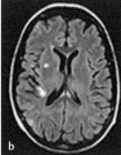

A. Total spine MRI
B. CT chest, abdomen, and pelvis
C. Gamma knife
D. Whole brain radiation

60.
Which of these metastatic tumor types has a higher risk of presenting with hemorrhage?

A. Lymphoma
B. Renal cell carcinoma
C. Squamous cell lung carcinoma
D. Ductal carcinoma in situ
E. Colon adenocarcinoma

61.
Which of these metastatic lesions is considered radiosensitive?

A. Multiple myeloma
B. Thyroid
C. Malignant melanoma
D. Renal cell carcinoma

62.
Which of these metastatic lesions is considered highly resistant to radiation?

A. Multiple myeloma
B. Breast cancer
C. Small cell lung cancer
D. Renal cell carcinoma

63.
What Karnofsky performance status score is a patient considered able to care for himself or herself without assistance?

A. 70
B. 80
C. 90
D. 100
E. 110

64.
You are evaluating a patient with a single, right frontal brain metastasis with no known primary who has a KPS of 100. What should you offer the patient?

A. Surgical resection
B. Gamma knife
C. Observation
D. Biopsy

65.
Primary CNS melanoma commonly arises from melanocytes located where?

A. Pachymeninges
B. Leptomeninges
C. Virchow-Robin spaces
D. Pia mater

66.

What percentage of incidentally discovered meningiomas will exhibit no growth over 3-year follow-up?

A. 10%
B. 33%
C. 66%
D. 90%
E. 100%

67.

Where do meningiomas arise from?

A. Oligodendrocytes
B. Arachnoid cap cells
C. Pachymeninges
D. Pia mater

68.

What is the overall incidence of meningiomas?

A. ~ 1 to 3%
B. ~ 8 to 10%
C. ~ 13 to 15%
D. ~ 18 to 20%
E. ~ 21 to 23%

69.

What is the most common location for a meningioma?

A. Sphenoid wing
B. Parasagittal
C. Convexity
D. Planum sphenoidale
E. Petrous apex

70.

Foster-Kennedy syndrome classically was caused by what tumor?

A. Medulloblastoma
B. Frontal glioblastoma
C. Olfactory groove meningioma
D. Clival chordoma

71.

What is the most common type of WHO grade II astrocytoma?

A. Anaplastic
B. Gemistocytic
C. Protoplasmic
D. Fibrillary

72.

What is considered the principal treatment for low-grade gliomas?

A. Observation
B. XRT alone
C. Chemotherapy + XRT
D. Surgical resection

73.

In patients with subtotally resected low-grade gliomas, early radiotherapy (54 Gy) has been associated with what results?

A. No difference in progression-free survival
B. 2-year increase in progression-free survival
C. 5-year increase in progression-free survival
D. 8-year increase in progression-free survival

74.

In patients with gross total resection of a low-grade glioma, early radiotherapy (54 Gy) has been associated with what results?

A. No difference in progression-free survival
B. 2-year increase in progression-free survival
C. 5-year increase in progression-free survival
D. 8-year increase in progression-free survival

75.

In patients with glioblastoma, what percentage of resection has been associated with increased overall survival?

A. > 50%
B. > 70%
C. > 85%
D. > 95%
E. > 97%

76.

The classic Stupp regimen of chemoradiation following glioblastoma resection consists of what?

A. 60 Gy XRT + PCV chemotherapy
B. 25 Gy XRT + temozolomide chemotherapy
C. 25 Gy XRT + PCV chemotherapy
D. 60 Gy XRT + temozolomide chemotherapy

77.

Giving 60 Gy XRT and temozolomide chemotherapy (Stupp) after resection of a glioblastoma is associated with a median overall survival of how many months?

A. 11.5 months
B. 14.6 months
C. 12.1 months
D. 18.3 months
E. 20.7 months

78.
MGMT promoter methylation in glioblastoma is associated with what median survival benefit compared to non-methylated tumors after utilization of the Stupp regimen of chemoradiation?

A. 6.3 months
B. 10.8 months
C. 23.4 months
D. 35.5 months
E. 40.2 months

79.
What is the main side effect of temozolomide chemotherapy?

A. Peripheral neuropathy
B. Myelosuppression
C. Cardiomyopathy
D. Leukocytosis
E. Seizures

80.
You are seeing a 55-year-old patient back in follow-up 3 months after a gross total resection of a glioblastoma of the right frontal lobe. She has undergone 60 Gy XRT and TMZ chemotherapy. Her tumor demonstrated MGMT promoter methylation. On her MRI there is evidence of a contrast enhancing nodule in the resection cavity. What is the likely cause of this finding?

A. Postoperative blood products
B. Tumor recurrence
C. Pseudoprogression
D. Ischemic stroke

81.
You are seeing a patient with recurrent glioblastoma who is currently undergoing treatment with bevacizumab (Avastin). All of the following are side effects of bevacizumab except?

A. Hypertension
B. Arterial thromboembolism
C. Hemorrhage
D. Myelosuppression

82.
Approximately 75% of pilocytic astrocytomas present in what age group?

A. 1 to 20 years
B. 21 to 40 years
C. 41 to 60 years
D. 61 to 80 years
E. 81 to 100 years

83.
What is the preferred postoperative treatment regimen for incompletely resected pilocytic astrocytomas in the pediatric population?

A. Observation
B. Early XRT
C. Temozolomide chemotherapy
D. Gamma knife

84.
Collins' law suggests that a pediatric patient with pilocytic astrocytomas can be considered cured if no recurrence happens in what time interval?

A. 5 years
B. 10 years
C. Patient's age at diagnosis + 5 years
D. Patient's age at diagnosis + 9 months

85.
A 16-year-old boy with a known history of NF-1 presents with painless proptosis. What is the most likely diagnosis?

A. Sphenoid wing meningioma
B. Optic glioma
C. Thyrotoxicosis
D. Orbital neurofibroma

86.
A 12-year-old girl presents with headache, nausea/vomiting, and diplopia. MRI is demonstrated below. What management should you recommend to the parents?

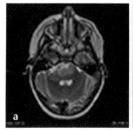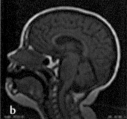

A. Surgical resection
B. Biopsy
C. Chemotherapy
D. Observation
E. Radiation

87.
Pleomorphic xanthoastrocytomas often present where?

A. Frontal lobe
B. Temporal lobe
C. Brainstem
D. Cerebellum
E. Occipital lobe

88.
You perform a subtotal resection of a tumor confirmed to be an oligodendroglioma based on final pathology. What is the recommended postoperative treatment?

A. 60 Gy XRT + temozolomide chemotherapy
B. 60 Gy XRT + PCV chemotherapy
C. PCV chemotherapy alone
D. Temozolomide chemotherapy alone

89.
You are evaluating a 33-year-old woman with what appears to be an ependymoma on MRI. If she were to present with a cranial nerve deficit, what deficit would you expect to see?

A. Visual loss
B. Medial rectus palsy
C. Facial weakness
D. Tongue weakness

90.
You are evaluating a 33-year-old woman with what appears to be an ependymoma on MRI of the brain. What other imaging should be performed?

A. Whole body PET CT
B. CT chest/abdomen/pelvis
C. MRI spinal axis
D. Technetium bone scan

91.
You resect an ependymoma of the fourth ventricle in a 33-year-old woman. MRI of the spinal axis does not demonstrate any evidence of drop metastases. What postoperative treatment would you recommend?

A. XRT + temozolomide chemotherapy
B. XRT + PCV chemotherapy
C. XRT alone
D. Temozolomide alone

92.
What tumor type is often found attached to the septum pellucidum?

A. Glioblastoma
B. Central neurocytoma
C. Intraventricular meningioma
D. Intraventricular lymphoma
E. Pleomorphic xanthoastrocytoma

93.
Gelastic seizures are often seen with a mass located where?

A. Frontal lobe
B. Mesial temporal lobe
C. Third ventricle
D. Anterior temporal pole
E. Fourth ventricle

94.
You have just resected a dysembryoplastic neuroepithelial tumor of the anterior temporal pole in a 22-year-old man with intractable epilepsy. Postoperative imaging suggests gross total resection. What do you recommend for postoperative management?

A. XRT + temozolomide chemotherapy
B. XRT alone
C. Temozolomide chemotherapy alone
D. Observation

95.
During surgery for a paraganglioma, manipulation of the tumor can lead to what intraoperative complication?

A. Cardiac arrhythmia
B. Life-threatening hemorrhage
C. Seizure
D. Stroke

96.
Which of the following is the most common type of paraganglioma?

A. Glomus tympanicum
B. Glomus jugulare
C. Glomus intravagale
D. Carotid body tumor

97.

Neuroblastomas arise from what element of the nervous system?

A. Sympathetic ganglion
B. Peripheral nerve
C. Dorsal root ganglion
D. Free nerve endings

98.

You are seeing a patient with a pineal region tumor. CSF markers are ordered and demonstrated below. What is the most likely diagnosis?

B-HCG (+), AFP (−), PLAP (−)

A. Germinoma
B. Choriocarcinoma
C. Embryonal carcinoma
D. Mature teratoma

99.

You are seeing a patient with a pineal region tumor. CSF markers are ordered and demonstrated below. What is the most likely diagnosis?

B-HCG (+), AFP (−), PLAP (+)

A. Germinoma
B. Choriocarcinoma
C. Embryonal carcinoma
D. Mature teratoma

100.

You are seeing a patient with a pineal region tumor. CSF markers are ordered and demonstrated below. What is the most likely diagnosis?

B-HCG (−), AFP (−), PLAP (−)

A. Germinoma
B. Choriocarcinoma
C. Embryonal carcinoma
D. Mature teratoma

101.

You are seeing a patient with a pineal region tumor. CSF markers are ordered and demonstrated below. What is the most likely diagnosis?

B-HCG (−), AFP (+), PLAP (−)

A. Germinoma
B. Choriocarcinoma
C. Embryonal carcinoma
D. Mature teratoma

102.

Patients with vestibular schwannomas are most likely to present with which of the symptoms listed below?

A. Facial weakness
B. Facial numbness
C. Taste changes
D. Otalgia

103.

What is the most common presentation of a vestibular schwannoma?

A. Facial weakness
B. Facial numbness
C. Taste changes
D. Hearing loss

104.

You see a 34-year-old woman with an asymptomatically discovered 1.3-cm vestibular schwannoma. Her hearing tests demonstrate intact hearing. What is the next best step?

A. Surgical resection
B. Stereotactic radiosurgery
C. Observation
D. Chemotherapy

105.

What direction is the facial nerve most often displaced by a vestibular schwannoma?

A. Anterior
B. Posterior
C. Superior
D. Inferior
E. Lateral

106.

What percentage of hemangioblastomas occur as part of von Hippel-Lindau disease?

A. 20%
B. 40%
C. 60%
D. 80%
E. 100%

107.

All of these tumor types are associated with von Hippel-Lindau disease except?

A. Hemangioblastoma
B. Pheochromocytoma
C. Paraganglioma
D. Renal cell carcinoma

108.
You are seeing a patient with biopsy proven, non-AIDS–related primary CNS lymphoma. What is the best treatment?
A. Surgical resection followed by XRT and methotrexate chemotherapy
B. XRT + methotrexate chemotherapy
C. XRT + temozolomide chemotherapy
D. Surgical resection followed by XRT and temozolomide chemotherapy

109.
What is the approximate 5-year survival of patients with biopsy proven primary CNS lymphoma?
A. 3 to 4%
B. 15 to 16%
C. 30 to 31%
D. 48 to 49%
E. 55 to 56%

110.
A pituitary tumor is considered a macroadenoma after it has crossed what size threshold?
A. > 5 mm
B. > 1 cm
C. > 2 cm
D. > 3 cm
E. > 3.5 cm

111.
Approximately what percentage of pituitary adenomas are functioning?
A. 15%
B. 35%
C. 50%
D. 65%
E. 80%

112.
What type of visual field deficit would a large pituitary macroadenoma cause?
A. Right homonymous hemianopia
B. Left superior quadrant hemianopia
C. Central scotoma
D. Bitemporal hemianopia

113.
What serum marker might help lead you to a diagnosis of suprasellar germinoma?
A. B-HCG
B. AFP
C. Sodium
D. Hematocrit

114.
You are taking care of a patient that you suspect has pituitary apoplexy. What finding would lead you to perform emergent decompression of the sella?
A. Hypotension
B. Visual field cut
C. Hypernatremia
D. Elevated urine output

115.
You see a patient with evidence of hypercortisolism. There appears to be a functioning pituitary adenoma. What is the diagnosis?
A. Cushing's disease
B. Cushing's syndrome
C. Nelson's syndrome
D. Pituitary apoplexy

116.
You are evaluating a patient who has had both adrenal glands removed as a treatment for her primary disease. She has noticed some worsening of her peripheral vision and states that her skin appears darker than usual. What is the diagnosis?
A. Cushing's disease
B. Cushing's syndrome
C. Nelson's syndrome
D. Pituitary apoplexy

117.
Patients with growth hormone-secreting pituitary adenomas have an elevated risk of what other type of cancer?
A. Lung cancer
B. Colon cancer
C. Pancreatic cancer
D. Hepatocellular carcinoma

118.
You see a patient with a large pituitary tumor and bitemporal hemianopia. Prolactin level is 356. You decide to attempt medical management. The main medication used in this case works on what receptor?
A. D1 dopamine receptor
B. D2 dopamine receptor
C. GABA receptor
D. Glutamate receptor

119.
You see a patient with a large pituitary tumor and bitemporal hemianopia. Prolactin level is 356. You decide to attempt medical management. You decide to use cabergoline. What is a worrisome side effect from the use of cabergoline?

A. Seizures
B. Diarrhea
C. Mitral regurgitation
D. Diabetes insipidus

120.
You are treating a patient with acromegaly and a growth hormone-secreting pituitary tumor. You elect to start the patient on medication using octreotide. How does this medication work?

A. GH receptor antagonist
B. Dopamine agonist
C. Somatostatin analogue
D. Adrenal steroid synthesis inhibitor

121.
You are treating a patient with acromegaly and a growth hormone-secreting pituitary tumor. You elect to start the patient on medication using pegvisomant. How does this medication work?

A. GH receptor antagonist
B. Dopamine agonist
C. Somatostatin analogue
D. Adrenal steroid synthesis inhibitor

122.
A patient presents to you with known colonic polyposis and evidence of multiple cranial osteomas in X-ray of the skull. What is the diagnosis?

A. Turcot's syndrome
B. Garnder's syndrome
C. McCune-Albright syndrome
D. Paget's disease

123.
You are seeing a patient with a single abnormal protrusion of the skull in the right parietal region. X-rays demonstrate trabeculated bone. They decide they would like it removed and during surgery you observe a blue colored mass underneath the pericranium. What is the most likely diagnosis?

A. Osteoid osteoma
B. Hemangioma
C. Metastasis
D. Multiple myeloma

124.
The Hand-Schüller-Christian triad is comprised of exophthalmos (from intraorbital tumor), lytic bone lesions (of the cranium), and what?

A. Diabetes insipidus
B. Seizures
C. Papilledema
D. Facial weakness

125.
Fibrous dysplasia is associated with what syndrome?

A. Turcot's syndrome
B. Garnder's syndrome
C. McCune-Albright syndrome
D. Paget's disease

126.
You are operating on a cerebellar hemangioblastoma with a large associated cystic component. You open the dura and the cerebellum begins to herniate through the dural defect. What will be the most effective means to decrease posterior fossa pressure?

A. Hyperventilation
B. Mannitol
C. Dexamethasone
D. Needle aspiration of cystic contents

127.
You resect a pathology proven cerebellar hemangioblastoma with a large cystic component. You have removed the mural nodule. Should you attempt to excise the entire cyst wall?

A. Yes
B. No

128.
You resect a pathology proven cerebellar pilocytic astrocytoma with a large cystic component. You have removed the mural nodule. Should you attempt to excise the entire cyst wall?

A. Yes
B. No

129.
During endoscopic third ventriculostomy, aggressive manipulation of the endoscope within the third ventricle should be avoided to prevent injury to what structure?

A. Mamillary bodies
B. Caudate head
C. Fornix
D. Thalamus

130.
Approximately what length of temporal lobe can be resected safely during a temporal lobectomy on the dominant side?

A. 1 to 2.5 cm
B. 3 to 4.5 cm
C. 5 to 5.5 cm
D. 6 to 6.5 cm

131.
You are seeing a patient in the emergency department who had the worst headache of her life. She opens her eyes to voice, does not know the date or where she is, but is able to follow commands reliably with good strength x4. Subarachnoid hemorrhage is confirmed on imaging. What is her WFNS grade?

A. 1
B. 2
C. 3
D. 4
E. 5

132.
You are seeing a patient in the emergency department who had the worst headache of her life. On imaging she has evidence of SAH in the basal cisterns that is >3 mm in diameter but no evidence of intra-ventricular hemorrhage. Based on the modified Fisher scale for SAH, what is her risk of vasospasm?

A. 0%
B. 24%
C. 33%
D. 40%
E. 50%

133.
After a ruptured intracranial aneurysm, what is the approximate risk of rebleed per day while the aneurysm remains unsecured?

A. 1.5%
B. 5%
C. 25%
D. 33%

134.
You are taking care of a patient who suffered a rupture of a carotid bifurcation aneurysm. It is postbleed day 5 and she is experiencing new left arm weakness. What is the most likely underlying mechanism?

A. Subclinical seizures
B. Hyponatremia
C. Vasospasm
D. Intracerebral hemorrhage

135.
What is the single most common location for an intracranial aneurysm?

A. Anterior communicating artery
B. Posterior communicating artery
C. Carotid bifurcation
D. Posterior inferior cerebellar artery

136.
You are evaluating a 55-year-old woman with a history of hypertension and smoking who has evidence of a third nerve palsy. Where is the aneurysm?

A. Anterior communicating artery
B. Posterior communicating artery
C. Carotid bifurcation
D. Posterior inferior cerebellar artery

137.
What is the most important step in aneurysm surgery prior to clip placement?

A. Dissecting the dome free
B. Releasing CSF
C. Proximal control
D. ICG administration

138.
You are seeing a patient with a right sided ophthalmic segment aneurysm that is growing and causing compression of the optic nerve from the aneurysm itself. What symptoms would you expect him to report?

A.   Right inferior nasal quadrantanopsia
B.   Right superior nasal quadrantanopsia
C.   Right superior temporal quadrantanopsia
D.   Right inferior temporal quadrantanopsia

139.
You are seeing a patient with a right sided ophthalmic segment aneurysm that is growing and causing compression of the optic nerve. This initially led to an ipsilateral superior nasal quadrantanopsia. Now he reports that he is developing an inferior nasal quadrantanopsia. What structure is causing further compression of the optic nerve?

A.   Falciform ligament
B.   Tuburculum sellae
C.   Anterior clinoid process
D.   Middle clinoid process

140.
You are seeing a patient with a right sided ophthalmic segment aneurysm that is growing and causing compression of the optic nerve. In order to gain access to the aneurysm neck you decide to perform an anterior clinoidectomy. What imaging modality might help you ensure that this procedure is safe in this patient's case?

A.   Conventional cerebral angiogram
B.   MRI brain
C.   CT head
D.   Carotid ultrasound

141.
You are evaluating an angiogram in a patient with an AVM. The characteristics are: size = 3.6 cm; drainage = internal cerebral vein; location = right frontal. What is the Spetzler-Martin grade of this AVM?

A.   2
B.   3
C.   4
D.   5
E.   6

142.
You are evaluating an angiogram in a patient with an AVM. The characteristics are: size = 3.6 cm; drainage = internal cerebral vein; location = right frontal. Based on Spetzler-Martin grade, what is the rate of good surgical outcome (no deficit postop)?

A.   95%
B.   84%
C.   73%
D.   69%
E.   53%

143.
What is the approximate annual risk of hemorrhage in S-M grade 1 to 3 AVMs?

A.   0%
B.   3.5%
C.   10%
D.   17.5%
E.   25%

144.
You are operating on a 35-year-old man with a brainstem cavernous malformation that has hemorrhaged twice. You successfully resect the cavernoma, but there appears to be a venous malformation deep in the resection cavity. True or false, you should coagulate and cut this venous malformation?

A.   True
B.   False

145.
You are operating on a 35-year-old man with a left temporal cavernous malformation that is thought to be causing his medically intractable epilepsy. As you approach to the cavernous malformation, you notice yellow discoloration of the surrounding brain parenchyma. True or false, you should resect this surrounding tissue?

A.   True
B.   False

146.
What is the most common presentation of a dural arteriovenous fistula?

A.   Hemorrhagic stroke
B.   Seizure
C.   Ischemic stroke
D.   Pulsatile tinnitus

147.

A Cognard grade II a + b dural arteriovenous fistula has what characteristic venous drainage?

A. Direct cortical venous drainage without ectasia
B. Direct cortical venous drainage with ectasia
C. Retrograde sinus and retrograde cortical venous drainage
D. Anterograde sinus and retrograde cortical venous drainage

148.

What Cognard grade carries the highest risk of hemorrhage when grading a dural fistula?

A. Type II a + b
B. Type III
C. Type II b
D. Type II a

149.

What is the most common presenting symptom of a vein of Galen malformation?

A. Hemorrhage
B. Seizure
C. Heart failure
D. Ischemic stroke

150.

You are evaluating a 44-year-old woman in the emergency department who was just involved in a motor vehicle accident where she was unrestrained and hit her face on the dashboard. Since the accident she has noticed blurry vision out of the right eye only. You notice that she appears to have a VI nerve palsy on the right, chemosis, and some proptosis. What is the diagnosis?

A. Intraparenchymal contusion
B. Orbital blowout fracture
C. Ophthalmic artery dissection
D. Carotid-cavernous fistula

151.

A hypoxic cell is more sensitive to radiation than an oxygenated cell, true or false?

A. True
B. False

152.

Generally speaking, how old should a child be before they are able to receive cranial radiation therapy?

A. > 1 year
B. > 3 years
C. > 5 years
D. > 7 years
E. > 10 years

153.

Gamma knife radiosurgery is used for tumors of what diameter?

A. 1 cm or less
B. 3 cm or less
C. 5 cm or less
D. 7 cm or less
E. 10 cm or less

154.

What is the maximum safe dose of radiation to the optic apparatus?

A. 6 Gy
B. 10 Gy
C. 14 Gy
D. 18 Gy
E. 20 Gy

155.

What is a standard stereotactic radiosurgery dose that gives good tumor control for vestibular schwannomas but preserves facial nerve function?

A. 10 Gy or less
B. 13 Gy or less
C. 16 Gy or less
D. 19 Gy or less
E. 22 Gy or less

156.

What is the maximum safe dose of radiation to the lens of the eye?

A. 6 Gy or less
B. 8 Gy or less
C. 10 Gy or less
D. 12 Gy or less
E. 15 Gy or less

157.

At the 10-year post-treatment mark, what percentage of patients who received standard sellar radiation for a residual pituitary tumor will experience side effects including hypopituitarism?

A. 10 to 20%
B. 20 to 30%
C. 30 to 40%
D. 40 to 50%
E. 50 to 60%

158.

What is considered the mean safe dose of radiation to the cochlea?

A. < 2 Gy
B. 4 to 6 Gy
C. 7 to 9 Gy
D. 10 to 12 Gy
E. 13 to 15 Gy

159.

You are seeing a 56-year-old man with a single brain metastasis which is proven to be a radio-sensitive tumor based on histology. You elect to perform stereotactic radiosurgery for this mass that measures approximately 1.8 cm in maximum diameter. What dose of radiation should you plan to deliver to the tumor?

A. 10 Gy
B. 18 Gy
C. 24 Gy
D. 30 Gy
E. 40 Gy

160.

You are seeing a 56-year-old man with a single brain metastasis which is proven to be a radio-sensitive tumor based on histology. You elect to perform stereotactic radiosurgery for this mass that measures approximately 2.8 cm in maximum diameter. What dose of radiation should you plan to deliver to the tumor?

A. 10 Gy
B. 18 Gy
C. 24 Gy
D. 30 Gy
E. 40 Gy

161.

You just resected a known, solitary lung cancer metastasis from the right frontal lobe in a 62-year-old man. Pathology confirms lung cancer metastasis. What is the next step for treatment?

A. Proton-beam radiation
B. Stereotactic radiosurgery
C. Whole brain radiation
D. Observation

162.

Current literature supports use of stereotactic radiosurgery to treat how many concurrent cerebral metastases?

A. 5 or less
B. 10 or less
C. 15 or less
D. 20 or less

163.

You are seeing a 34-year-old woman with a Spetzler-Martin grade II AVM (2.8 cm nidus, borders eloquent cortex), and she prefers stereotactic radiosurgery as an initial attempt at treating her currently asymptomatic AVM. She asks you how long it takes for the radiation to close the AVM. You tell her…

A. < 1 week
B. < 1 month
C. < 1 year
D. < 3 years
E. > 5 years

164.

You are seeing a 34-year-old woman with a Spetzler-Martin grade II AVM (2.8 cm nidus, borders eloquent cortex), and she prefers stereotactic radiosurgery as an initial attempt at treating her currently asymptomatic AVM. What radiation dose should you administer to the AVM?

A. 14 to 16 Gy
B. 18 to 20 Gy
C. 23 to 25 Gy
D. 29 to 31 Gy

165.
What is the overall AVM obliteration rate when treated by stereotactic radiosurgery?

A. 10 to 20%
B. 30 to 40%
C. 50 to 60%
D. 70 to 80%
E. 90 to 100%

166.
What is the approximate "pain-free" control rate of trigeminal neuralgia when treated by stereotactic radiosurgery?

A. 25%
B. 45%
C. 65%
D. 85%

167.
What is the primary deleterious side effect of whole brain radiation?

A. Intracerebral hemorrhage
B. Seizures
C. Headaches
D. Dementia

168.
You are evaluating a patient in the emergency department with known multiple myeloma who is presenting with signs and symptoms of spinal cord compression. Imaging confirms an epidural mass emanating from the vertebral body. You call a colleague in radiation oncology and she says she can administer emergency radiation to shrink the tumor. Approximately what dose will she deliver in this situation?

A. 8 Gy
B. 15 Gy
C. 22 Gy
D. 30 Gy

169.
What is the standard radiation dose administered to the spine for metastatic disease?

A. 10 Gy in 10 fractions
B. 20 Gy in 10 fractions
C. 30 Gy in 10 fractions
D. 40 Gy in 10 fractions

170.
You are seeing a 55-year-old woman with severe right sided trigeminal neuralgia currently on carbamazepine that is currently controlled. What percentage of patients managed with medication will ultimately require a procedure?

A. 5%
B. 50%
C. 75%
D. 100%

171.
During a microvascular decompression, you do not see a compressive vessel and you elect to squeeze the nerve. What is a significant risk of performing this procedure?

A. Anesthesia dolorosa
B. Worsened facial pain
C. Brainstem ischemic stroke
D. Seizure

172.
You are seeing a 55-year-old woman who reports pain in her lower right jaw and teeth. It seems lancinating in nature and brought on by brushing her teeth. She has lost weight because she finds it difficult to eat. What should be your next step?

A. Start carbamazepine
B. MRI brain with FIESTA sequences
C. Right sided microvascular decompression
D. Observation

173.
You are seeing a 55-year-old woman who reports pain in her lower right jaw and teeth. It seems lancinating in nature and brought on by brushing her teeth. She has lost weight because she finds it difficult to eat. What should be your next step?

A. Start carbamazepine
B. Start oxycodone
C. Right sided microvascular decompression
D. Right sided percutaneous trigeminal rhizotomy

174.
What is the success rate of microvascular decompression at 10 years?

A. 30%
B. 50%
C. 70%
D. 90%

175.
How do you determine the difference between SIADH and cerebral salt wasting?

A. Urine osmolality
B. Serum sodium
C. Fluid status
D. Urine output

176.
What is an initial step for treating SIADH and hyponatremia in a patient who is conscious and able to follow commands?

A. Hypertonic saline
B. Fluid restriction
C. DDAVP
D. Demeclocycline

177.
You are treating a patient with SIADH refractory to fluid restriction. You decide to utilize medical management. What medication should you start?

A. Furosemide
B. Hydrocortisone
C. DDAVP
D. Demeclocycline

178.
You are treating a patient with cerebral salt wasting refractory to fluid resuscitation. You decide to utilize medical management. What medication should you start?

A. Furosemide
B. Fludrocortisone
C. DDAVP
D. Demeclocycline

179.
What is an initial step for treating cerebral salt wasting and hyponatremia in a patient with subarachnoid hemorrhage?

A. Normal saline infusion
B. Fluid restriction
C. DDAVP
D. Demeclocycline

180.
Untreated diabetes insipidus leads to what medical condition?

A. Hyponatremia
B. Severe dehydration
C. Coma
D. Status epilepticus

181.
How much secretory capacity for ADH must be lost before central diabetes insipidus occurs?

A. 25%
B. 55%
C. 85%
D. 100%

182.
You are taking care of a conscious, ambulatory patient with mild diabetes insipidus. How should you manage the patient's sodium?

A. Drink to thirst
B. DDAVP administration
C. Salt tablets
D. Hypertonic saline infusion

183.
At what dose does the use of a dopamine infusion become a vasoconstrictor rather than a positive inotrope?

A. > 2 µg/kg/min
B. > 5 µg/kg/min
C. > 10 µg/kg/min
D. > 15 µg/kg/min

184.
You elect to use dobutamine to increase the cardiac output of one of your postop patients. How long will this medication be effective?

A. 12 hours
B. 24 hours
C. 48 hours
D. 72 hours

185.
How long can an outpatient be on steroids before you should consider starting GI (ulcer) prophylaxis?

A. < 2 days
B. < 1 week
C. < 3 weeks
D. < 6 months
E. 1 year

186.
One unit of platelets (out of a "six pack") is expected to raise the platelet count by approximately how much?

A. 1 to 5K
B. 5 to 10K
C. 10 to 15K
D. 15 to 20K

187.
What platelet count should cause you to transfuse platelets even in the setting of no evidence of bleeding?

A. 10K
B. 30K
C. 50K
D. 75K

188.
What is the dose for reversing unfractionated heparin utilizing protamine sulfate?

A. 1 mg protamine/10 u heparin
B. 1 mg protamine/100 u heparin
C. 1 mg protamine/1,000 u heparin
D. 1 mg protamine/10,000 u heparin

189.
You see a stable patient with a subdural hematoma who is on Dabigatran (Pradaxa). In order to reverse the anticoagulation you elect to give Idarucizumab (Praxbind). How long should you wait before proceeding to the operating room?

A. Immediately
B. 4 hours
C. 12 hours
D. 24 hours

190.
You are evaluating a post-operative craniotomy patient in the PACU. The anesthesia team utilized succinylcholine during intubation. The patient appears to be tachypneic, tachycardia, severe rigidity and high fever. What is the likely diagnosis?

A. Hyperkalemia
B. Seizure
C. Malignant hyperthermia
D. Respiratory failure

191.
You are evaluating a postoperative craniotomy patient in the PACU. The anesthesia team utilized succinylcholine during intubation. The patient appears to be tachypneic, tachycardic, with severe rigidity and high fever. What medication should be administered?

A. Benzodiazepines
B. Propofol
C. Dantrolene
D. Desmopressin

192.
You are evaluating a postoperative craniotomy patient in the PACU. The anesthesia team utilized succinylcholine during intubation. The patient appears to be tachypneic, tachycardic, with severe rigidity and high fever. This condition is thought to arise from genetic defects in what receptor?

A. Nicotinic
B. Ryanodine
C. NMDA
D. GABA

193.
Based on the NASCET study, what is the reduction in stroke risk after carotid endarterectomy in symptomatic patients with high grade stenosis at 18 months post-procedure compared to best medical management?

A. 6%
B. 11%
C. 17%
D. 23%
E. 28%

194.
Based on the current literature, what should the overall risk of postoperative complications be to justify a carotid endarterectomy for a patient with symptomatic high-grade stenosis?

A. 1% or less
B. 3% or less
C. 5% or less
D. 7% or less
E. 10% or less

195.
You are evaluating a patient in the PACU in whom you just performed a left sided carotid endarterectomy. She reports that she has had two episodes since surgery of her usual amaurosis fugax TIA. Her neck is not enlarged. What is the next best step?

A. EEG
B. CT angiogram
C. MRI
D. Bedside decompression

196.
You are evaluating a patient in the ICU in whom you just performed a left-sided carotid endarterectomy approximately 12 hours ago. She reports that she has a fairly severe left-sided headache and her left eye hurts. What next step will most likely improve her symptoms?

A. Pain medication administration
B. CT angiogram
C. Blood pressure control
D. Operative exploration

197.
What is the most common cranial neuropathy to occur after carotid endarterectomy?

A. Hypoglossal palsy
B. Spinal accessory palsy
C. Vagus palsy
D. Glossopharyngeal palsy

198.
You are called emergently to the PACU to evaluate a post-operative carotid endarterectomy patient who is having trouble breathing. She has obvious stridor and her saturations are dropping. She appears to have a bulging mass in the operative site. What should you do?

A. CT Angiogram
B. Bedside decompression
C. Intubation
D. Oxygen administration

199.
You are evaluating a patient who just experienced a stroke with a small fixed deficit and evidence of high grade stenosis of the left carotid artery. You elect to offer a carotid endarterectomy. This procedure should be performed within what timeframe from the stroke onset to improve outcome?

A. 1 week
B. 2 weeks
C. 3 weeks
D. 1 month

200.
The carotid revascularization endarterectomy versus stenting trial demonstrated what when comparing the outcomes of carotid angioplasty and stenting to carotid endarterectomy?

A. Superiority
B. Nonsuperiority
C. Inferiority
D. Noninferiority
E. Worsened outcomes

2 Neurology

1.
You are evaluating a 56-year-old woman who had the onset of midthoracic back pain which has progressed to quadriparesis over the last several days. She has also noted the onset of bilateral severe eye pain and is losing vision in the left eye based on your visual acuity exam. Her imaging is demonstrated below. The underlying pathophysiology of this condition is thought to arise due to auto-antibodies against what?

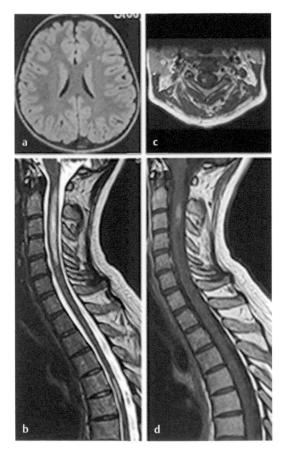

A.   T lymphocytes
B.   Aquaporin channel
C.   Myelin
D.   Presynaptic calcium channel
E.   Postsynaptic acetylcholine channel

2.
You are evaluating a 33-year-old woman with AIDS who has the following imaging. She has headaches, mild vision loss, and ataxia. What is the underlying cause of this patient's condition?

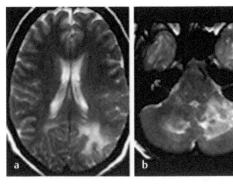

A.   BK virus infection
B.   Amoeba infection
C.   HIV virus infection
D.   JC virus infection
E.   Toxoplasmosis

3.
Ciliary paralysis is seen in what condition listed below?

A.   Myasthenia gravis
B.   Botulism
C.   AIDP
D.   CIDP
E.   PML

4.
You are evaluating a patient in the emergency department that has an interesting neurologic finding on examination. When you ask the patient to look up, his eyes converge and retract in a bilateral jerk-movement fashion. The lesion is most likely located where?

A.   Ventral midbrain
B.   Dorsal pons
C.   Dorsal midbrain
D.   Ventral pons
E.   Hypothalamus

5.

In a patient with a hypertensive hemorrhage of the pons, what exam finding would you expect?

A. Mydriasis
B. Bilateral third nerve palsy
C. Productive aphasia
D. Miosis
E. Expressive aphasia

6.

What neuron must be intact for amphetamine (Paredrine) to affect pupillary size?

A. First order neuron
B. Second order neuron
C. Third order neuron
D. Fourth order neuron
E. Fifth order neuron

7.

Friedrich's ataxia is inherited in what fashion?

A. Autosomal recessive
B. Autosomal dominant
C. X-linked recessive
D. Sporadic
E. Autosomal dominant with incomplete penetrance

8.

The following MRI finding is often demonstrated in what inherited condition?

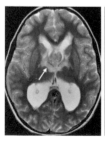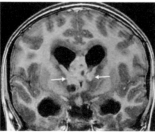

A. Neurofibromatosis type I
B. Neurofibromatosis type II
C. Sturge-Weber disease
D. Tuberous sclerosis
E. VHL

9.

In many patients with HIV that go on to develop intracranial primary lymphoma, what is thought to be the underlying causative mechanism and type of lymphoma?

A. Epstein-Barr virus/T cell type
B. Epstein-Barr virus/B cell type
C. JC virus/T cell type
D. JC virus/B cell type
E. BK virus/B cell type

10.

What protein is found in Alzheimer's-associated neurofibrillary tangles?

A. Amyloid
B. Ubiquitin
C. Tau protein
D. Alpha-synuclein
E. APOE e4

11.

In patients with advanced Alzheimer's dementia, neurofibrillary tangles and plaques seen in what region are associated with the highest grade of dementia?

A. Substantia nigra
B. CA1 hippocampus
C. Ventral medulla
D. Occipital cortex
E. Corpus callosum

12.

You are evaluating a 5-year-old boy who has had difficulty with walking since age 3. He has a waddling gait and has difficulty standing due to proximal muscle weakness. A muscle biopsy is demonstrated below. What gene is affected?

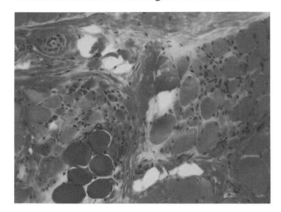

A. Emerin/completely absent
B. Emerin/partial dysfunction
C. Dystrophin/completely absent
D. Dystrophin/partial dysfunction
E. Myotonin/completely absent

13.

Which autoantibody is found in patients with limbic encephalitis?

A. Anti-Hu
B. Anti-Yo
C. Anti-Ri
D. Anti-glutamic acid decarboxylase
E. Anti-Ma

14.

You are asked to evaluate a high school football player on the sideline of his football game where he was hit hard on the helmet and appears confused. The brain dysfunction seen during the acute post-concussive syndrome is thought to arise due to what process?

A. Axon disruption
B. Subclinical seizures
C. ATP pump failure
D. Neurotransmitter depletion
E. Excitatory toxicity

15.

What is the best initial management of post-concussive syndrome?

A. Immediate return to play
B. Cognitive rest
C. Prophylactic antiepileptic medications
D. Opioid pain medications
E. Intensive blood pressure management

16.

You are evaluating a pediatric patient who is thought to have Rasmussen's encephalitis, resulting from chronic encephalitis with spreading cortical inflammation. This results in epilepsy partialis continua. What is a common treatment technique in these patients?

A. VA nucleus DBS
B. Functional hemispherectomy
C. Medical management
D. Vagal nerve stimulator
E. Motor cortex stimulator

17.

You are rotating in the EEG department and see a patient with the following EEG. What is the best medication for this patient?

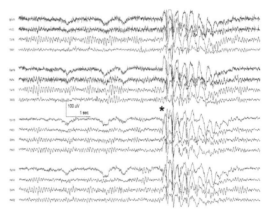

A. Valproic acid
B. Carbamazepine
C. Ethosuxamide
D. Levetiracetam
E. Zonisamide

18.

What percentage of patients with an uncomplicated, simple febrile seizure will go on to develop adult epilepsy?

A. < 5%
B. 15%
C. 25%
D. 35%
E. 50%

19.

The following MRI demonstrates findings associated with what syndrome?

A. Hemimegalencephaly
B. Focal cortical dysplasia
C. Joubert syndrome
D. Lhermitte-Duclos syndrome
E. Rhombencephalosynapsis

20.

How do patients with postoperative brachial neuritis (Parsonage-Turner syndrome) present?

A. Pain before weakness
B. Weakness before pain
C. Weakness alone
D. Pain alone
E. Hyperreflexia alone

21.

In patients with the following finding, what syndrome should you suspect?

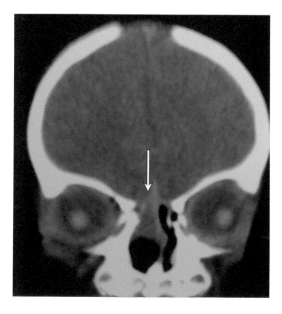

A. Sturge-Weber syndrome
B. Neurofibromatosis type I
C. Blue rubber bleb nevus syndrome
D. Ataxia telangiectasia
E. Friedrich's ataxia

22.

You see a patient on rounds that appears to have transverse white lines on her fingernails, also known as Mees' lines. What toxic exposure are these signs associated with?

A. Lead
B. Arsenic
C. Mercury
D. Strychnine
E. Botulinum toxin

23.

A patient with a PTEN mutation may be found to have what underlying process?

A. Dysembryoplastic gangliocytoma of the cerebellum
B. Optic glioma
C. Brainstem cavernous malformation
D. Butterfly glioma
E. Multiple meningiomas

24.

Patients with narcolepsy exhibit onset of what sleep stage immediately upon falling asleep?

A. Stage II sleep
B. Stage IV sleep
C. REM sleep
D. Stage I sleep
E. Stage III sleep

25.

When reading an EEG, what electrode corresponds to the right frontal region?

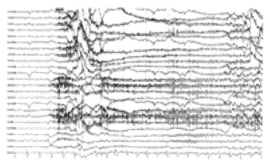

A. F1
B. F2
C. C3
D. C4
E. O2

26.

Cheyne Stokes respirations are thought to arise from destruction of what brain region?

A. Medullary destruction
B. Pontine destruction
C. Bifrontal destruction
D. Bithalamic destruction
E. Pontomedullary destruction

27.

Nelson's syndrome describes what process after bilateral adrenalectomy?

A. Pituitary adenoma enlargement
B. Panhypopituitarism
C. Pituitary apoplexy
D. Spontaneous CSF leak
E. Optic chiasm compression in nonfunctioning pituitary adenomas

28.

The patient with the findings depicted in this image would have what findings on laboratory evaluation?

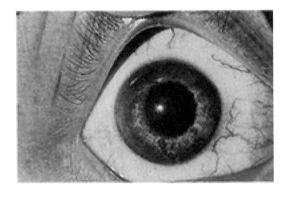

A. Low serum ceruloplasmin, high urine copper
B. High serum ceruloplasmin, high urine copper
C. Low serum ceruloplasmin, low urine copper
D. High serum ceruloplasmin, low urine copper

29.

You are preparing to perform a C6-7 ACDF on a patient with a single-level traumatic jumped facet. You elect to utilize MEP and SSEP monitoring for the case. Before making incision, the monitoring technician informs you that there is prolonged latency of the ulnar SSEPs at Erb's point on the right. What is the most likely cause of this change?

A. Spinal cord compression
B. Positioning-related brachial plexus compression
C. Intracranial hemorrhage, parietal cortex
D. Spinal cord vascular compromise
E. Intracranial hemorrhage, thalamus

30.

A diabetic third nerve palsy is often?

A. Painful and permanent
B. Painful and temporary
C. Painless and permanent
D. Painless and temporary

31.

You are evaluating a 32-year-old woman who reports ongoing difficulties with severe, burning pain of the right upper extremity. She has no history of trauma to the extremity. It appears red and warm, and she will not let you touch the extremity due to significant allodynia. She has not had good benefit from medical management. What is another potential treatment for her pain?

A. Limb amputation
B. Sensory neurectomy
C. Percutaneous cordotomy
D. Sympathetic blockade
E. Cervical laminectomy

32.

You are evaluating a 44-year-old man who developed a sudden headache and speech difficulty. His imaging is demonstrated below. What condition might this patient have?

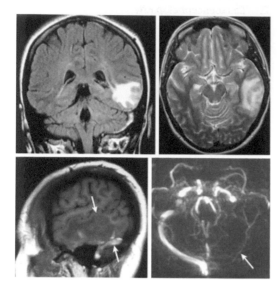

A. Neurofibromatosis
B. AIDS
C. Homocystinuria
D. Phenylketonuria
E. Blue rubber bleb nevus syndrome

33.

You have a patient in burst suppression on pentobarbital for elevated ICP. You decide to turn off the pentobarbital now in order to get a neuro exam. Approximately how long will you have to wait for return of neurological function?

A. 5 hours
B. 24 hours
C. 48 hours
D. 72 hours
E. 100+ hours

34.

You are evaluating the EMG of a patient in whom there is an intact F wave, but the H-reflex is absent. Where is the injury most likely located?

A. Motor endplate
B. Distal motor nerve
C. Dorsal root ganglion
D. Upper cervical spine
E. Anterior horn cells

35.

Which of the following findings would help you to determine whether a patient has zoster oticus or Bell's palsy?

A. Upper facial weakness
B. Lower facial weakness
C. Ear vesicles
D. Facial pain
E. Corneal abrasion

36.

You are asked to see an 86-year-old woman who reports dizziness. She says she hasn't really had this before the last 2 days and it seemed to start all of a sudden. She has had difficulty standing and walking due to the dizziness. On exam she has spontaneous, direction changing nystagmus and skew deviation. She reports minimal nausea and no vomiting since onset. What is the next best step in management?

A. Scopolamine patch
B. Otolith repositioning
C. Antibiotics
D. Brain MRI
E. Dexamethasone

37.

What structure of the auditory system is most sensitive to high volume?

A. Tympanic membrane
B. Inner hair cells
C. Outer hair cells
D. Semicircular canals
E. Spiral ganglion

38.
Internuclear ophthalmoplegia affects what brain-stem tract?

A. Medial longitudinal fasciculus
B. Paramedian pontine reticular formation
C. Corticospinal tract
D. Rubrospinal tract
E. Optic tract

39.
Bilateral carpal tunnel syndrome would be classified as what?

A. Polyradiculopathy
B. Mononeuropathy
C. Mononeuropathy multiplex
D. Polyneuropathy
E. Peripheral neuropathy

40.
What would you expect to see on EMG of a patient with Lambert-Eaton syndrome?

A. Decremental response
B. Incremental response
C. Steady response
D. No response

41.
This MRI demonstrates lesions discovered in a 29-year-old man with known AIDS. What is the diagnosis?

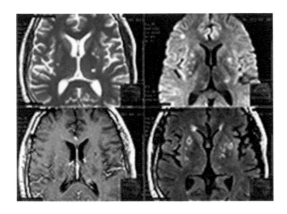

A. HIV encephalopathy
B. Staph aureus abscess
C. Listeria abscess
D. Toxoplasmosis
E. PML

42.
What is the most common neurologic complication in patients with AIDS?

A. Toxoplasmosis
B. Primary lymphoma
C. Leukoencephalopathy
D. Bacterial abscess
E. Glioma

43.
Charcot joints are thought to be due to what process?

A. Obesity
B. Peripheral neuropathy
C. Complex regional pain syndrome
D. Infection
E. Tumor

44.
A patient who demonstrates the opsoclonus-myoclonus reaction (rapid, involuntary conjugate eye movements in multiple directions associated with myoclonic jerks) may have which of the following tumors?

A. Glioblastoma
B. Hemangioblastoma
C. Neuroblastoma
D. Pineoblastoma
E. Choroid plexus carcinoma

45.
You see a pediatric patient who suffers from intractable epilepsy that manifests as drop attacks. He has had several injuries related to his seizures. What surgical procedure might provide him some relief from his condition?

A. Functional hemispherectomy
B. Corpus callosotomy
C. Temporal lobectomy
D. Selective amygdalohippocampectomy

46.

You are evaluating a child on the pediatric neurology service that is currently hospitalized for a subdural hematoma. He appears to have kinked hair, and laboratory studies have demonstrated low levels of ceruloplasmin. What is the inheritance pattern of this disorder?

A. X-linked
B. Autosomal dominant
C. Sporadic
D. Autosomal recessive

47.

The term "palinopsia" refers to what symptom?

A. Color blindness
B. Inability to recognize faces
C. Burned in images when eyes are closed
D. Cortical blindness
E. Visual field cut

48.

The following findings are often seen in patients with what genetic condition?

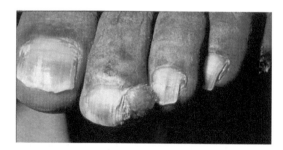

A. NF1
B. NF2
C. Sturge-Weber syndrome
D. Blue rubber bleb nevus syndrome
E. Tuberous sclerosis

49.

You evaluate a patient with macrocephaly, developmental delay, and seizures. He is an infant. MR imaging demonstrates bifrontal symmetric T2 hyperintensities. There is concern for Alexander disease. If a brain biopsy were to be performed, what would you expect to see on pathology?

A. Hirano bodies
B. Rosenthal fibers
C. Lewy bodies
D. Neurofibrillary tangles
E. Eosinophilic cytoplasmic inclusion bodies

50.

Which of the following is not a part of Wernicke's triad?

A. Ataxia
B. Ophthalmoplegia
C. Confusion
D. Aphasia

3 Neuroanatomy

1.

The medial posterior choroidal artery originates from which segment of the posterior cerebral artery?

A. P1
B. P2
C. P3
D. P4

2.

While performing an anterior temporal lobectomy, your medial resection ends at the ambient cistern. What cranial nerve passes through this space?

A. Trigeminal
B. Oculomotor
C. Trochlear
D. Optic

3.

The vidian artery originates from which segment of the internal carotid artery?

A. Cavernous
B. Lacerum
C. Ophthalmic
D. Petrous

4.

While operating on an anterior convexity meningioma, you attempt to obtain negative margins around the tumor. What structure do you need to disconnect the falx from to ensure a clean inferior margin?

A. Crista galli
B. Anterior clinoid
C. Orbital roof
D. Sphenoid ridge

5.

Brodmann area 17 is supplied by which artery?

A. Superior cerebellar artery
B. Callosal marginal artery
C. Calcarine artery
D. Splenial artery

6.

Brodmann area 44 corresponds to which cortical region?

A. Precentral gyrus
B. Inferior frontal gyrus
C. Gyrus rectus
D. Middle frontal gyrus

7.

The lentiform nucleus is comprised of which structures?

A. Caudate and putamen
B. Putamen and globus pallidus
C. Caudate and globus pallidus
D. Primary motor cortex and putamen

8.

The claustrum separates which two structures?

A. Putamen and external capsule
B. Extreme capsule and insular cortex
C. Globus pallidus and internal capsule
D. External capsule and extreme capsule

9.

While assessing a patient after a stroke, your exam identifies a pure conductive aphasia. Which structure has been damaged?

A. Arcuate fasciculus
B. Broca's area
C. Wernicke's area
D. Primary motor cortex

10.

While clipping a posterior communicating artery aneurysm, the clip is inadvertently placed across an artery in the region. What postoperative deficit would not be expected after ligation of this artery?

A. Contralateral hemiparesis
B. Contralateral hemisensory loss
C. Contralateral hemianopia
D. Ipsilateral monocular blindness

11.

During exposure of an anterior communicating artery aneurysm, you decide to drain CSF directly from the third ventricle. In order to do this, you perforate a structure just posterior to the optic chiasm. This structure is formed on which day of embryologic development?

A. Day 22
B. Day 24
C. Day 26
D. Day 28

12.

Which of the following is the correct association of a thalamic nucleus and its corresponding cortical projections?

A. Pulvinar–Cingulate gyrus
B. Anterior nuclei–Orbital frontal cortex and frontal eye fields
C. Mediodorsal nuclei–Primary and secondary visual cortices
D. Ventral posterolateral nuclei–Somatosensory cortex

13.

Which hippocampal region is most resistant to hypoxia?

A. CA1
B. CA2
C. CA3
D. CA4

14.

The main artery feeding the pachymeninges enters the skull through which foramen?

A. Foramen spinosum
B. Foramen lacerum
C. Foramen ovale
D. Foramen rotundum

15.

In the roof of the third ventricle, where are the fornices in relation to the internal cerebral veins?

A. Medial
B. Superior
C. Lateral
D. Inferior

16.

Through what structure does the hypothalamus receive projections from the hippocampus?

A. Medial forebrain bundle
B. Fornix
C. Stria terminalis
D. Inferior longitudinal fasciculus

17.

What is the largest input to the amygdala?

A. Locus ceruleus
B. Ventral tegmentum
C. Nucleus basalis of Meynert
D. Insular cortex

18.

Primary input to Brodmann areas 41 and 42 come from which region?

A. Medial geniculate body
B. Lateral geniculate body
C. Inferior colliculus
D. Superior colliculus

19.

You have been following a patient with epilepsy. Her seizure semiology consists of olfactory hallucinations followed by behavioral arrest, lip smacking and left upper extremity shaking. You offer surgical resection for attempted cure. What deficit is possible in this case if resection is carried too far posterior?

A. Right hemiplegia
B. Left hemiplegia
C. Left superior quadrantanopsia
D. Left inferior quadrantanopsia

20.

A 60-year-old man has bradykinesia, rigidity and impaired balance. You are performing a DBS electrode placement to the most commonly targeted nuclei that improve rigidity in this disorder. During test stimulation of the electrode, the patient develops ipsilateral eye deviation. Which direction should you move the electrode?

A. Lateral
B. Medial
C. Superior
D. Inferior

21.

You are performing bilateral STN DBS for a patient with advanced Parkinsonism. During test stimulation, the patient develops contralateral facial pulling and contralateral arm twitching. Which direction should you move the electrode?

A. Anteromedial
B. Posteromedial
C. Anterolateral
D. Posterolateral

22.

You are performing DBS electrode placement for dystonia. While targeting the most common nuclei for this disorder, the patient develops contralateral muscle contractions, which direction do you need to move the electrode?

A. Lateral
B. Medial
C. Anterior
D. Posterior

23.

During a DBS lead placement for dystonia, your patient develops phosphenes in her visual field during test stimulation, which direction should you move the electrode?

A. Inferior
B. Superior
C. Medial
D. Lateral

24.

You are placing DBS electrodes in a 45-year-old man who has been diagnosed with essential tremor. While targeting the most common nuclei for this disorder, your patient develops muscle contractions during test stimulation. Which direction should you move the electrode?

A. Inferior
B. Superior
C. Medial
D. Lateral

25.

While placing DBS electrodes for essential tremor into VIM thalamus, the patient develops persistent paresthesias during test stimulation. Which direction should you move the electrode?

A. Anterior
B. Posterior
C. Medial
D. Lateral

26.

You are exposing a right sided ICA terminus aneurysm for surgical clipping. You decide to dissect along the MCA (M1 segment) to reach the ICA terminus and the aneurysm. Which area of the M1 segment of the MCA is considered safe?

A. Posterosuperior
B. Posteroinferior
C. Anterosuperior
D. Anteroinferior

27.

This structure connects the temporal and orbital cortical regions. Medially it is bordered by the anterior perforated substance. Laterally it is bordered by the insular cortex.

A. Medial forebrain bundle
B. Limen insulae
C. Inferior longitudinal fasciculus
D. Diagonal band of Broca

28.

You are performing an anterior interhemispheric approach to the third ventricle for a presumed teratoma. In order to expose the corpus callosum for division, you must retract the cortex. What is the gyrus located immediately superior to the corpus callosum.

A. Cingulate gyrus
B. Paracentral lobule
C. Supramarginal gyrus
D. Precentral gyrus

29.

Which vein does not drain directly into the great cerebral vein of Galen?

A. Precentral cerebellar vein
B. Basal vein of Rosenthal
C. Internal cerebral vein
D. Thalamostriate vein

30.

You are performing an ETV on a pediatric patient for congenital acqueductal stenosis. You are looking at the floor of the third ventricle and you have identified the mammillary bodies. Which direction in relation to the mammillary bodies is the safe zone for puncture?

A. Anterior
B. Lateral
C. Posterior
D. Medial

31.

In the anterior floor of the third ventricle, what structure is located just above the supraoptic recess?

A. Anterior commissure
B. Lamina terminalis
C. Optic chiasm
D. Mammillary bodies

32.

Descending laterally across the posterior skull, which suture marks the border between the occipital and parietal bones?

A. Squamosal
B. Coronal
C. Lambdoid
D. Sphenosquamosal

33.
Which sutures connect to form the bregma?

A. Sagittal-lambdoid
B. Parietomastoid-occipitomastoid
C. Squamosal-parietomastoid
D. Coronal-sagittal

34.
Which structure is not part of the deep cerebellar nuclei?

A. Globose
B. Fastigial
C. Emboliform
D. Vestibular

35.
Which structure forms the superolateral border of the 4th ventricle?

A. Brachium conjunctivum
B. Restiform body
C. Brachium pontis
D. Vermis

36.
Which structure forms the inferolateral border of the 4th ventricle?

A. Brachium conjunctivum
B. Restiform body
C. Brachium pontis
D. Vermis

37.
Which cerebellar lobe forms what is considered to be the functional cerebellar division known as the vestibulocerebellum?

A. Anterior lobe
B. Posterior lobe
C. Vermis
D. Flocculonodular lobe

38.
Which cerebellar region forms what is considered to be the functional cerebellar division known as the cerebrocerebellum?

A. Anterior lobe
B. Lateral hemisphere
C. Vermis
D. Flocculonodular lobe

39.
Which cerebellar region forms what is considered to be the functional cerebellar division known as the spinocerebellum?

A. Anterior lobe
B. Lateral hemisphere
C. Vermis
D. Flocculonodular lobe

40.
What is the primary output of the paramedian pontine reticular formation (PPRF)?

A. Trochlear nucleus
B. Abducens nucleus
C. Oculomotor nucleus
D. Facial nucleus

41.
You are evaluating a patient with double vision. When you are testing external ocular movements, the right eye fails to adduct when you attempt to make the patient track your finger to the patient's left. What structure is likely damaged?

A. Right abducens nerve
B. Medial longitudinal fasciculus
C. Left abducens nerve
D. Medial lemniscus

42.
After resecting a 4th ventricular subependymoma, you are viewing the floor of the 4th ventricle. You notice bilateral raised circular structures. What is the most likely structure that you notice?

A. Trochlear nuclei
B. Facial colliculus
C. Stria medullaris
D. Middle cerebellar peduncle

43.
On the floor of the 4th ventricle, the vagal trigone is located where in relation to the hypoglossal trigone?

A. Medial
B. Lateral
C. Superior
D. Inferior

44.

Myelinated neurons from the nucleus gracilis and nucleus cuneatus decussate in the medulla to form the medial lemniscus. What are the decussating connections called?

A. Medial longitudinal fasciculus
B. Internal arcuate fibers
C. Pyramids
D. Mossy fibers

45.

What is the only paired circumventricular organ?

A. Area prostrema
B. Subforniceal organ
C. Vascular organ of the lamina terminalis
D. Subcommissural organ

46.

Within the cerebral peduncles, the descending corticospinal tract fibers controlling sacral function are located where?

A. Medially
B. Anteriorly
C. Laterally
D. Posteriorly

47.

The oculomotor nucleus is located at which horizontal level within the brainstem?

A. Cerebral peduncles
B. Superior colliculi
C. Inferior colliculi
D. Pons

48.

Which nucleus is the center of control for the direct and consensual pupillary light reflex?

A. Interstitial nucleus of Cajal
B. Oculomotor
C. Pretectal
D. Trochlear

49.

What is the only circumventricular organ to have an intact blood brain barrier?

A. Subcommissural organ
B. Subforniceal organ
C. Area prostrema
D. Pineal gland

50.

What structure is located lateral to the red nucleus within the midbrain?

A. IIIrd nerve fibers
B. Periacqueductal grey
C. Medial longitudinal fasciculus
D. Medial lemniscus

51.

Which artery provides the majority of blood supply to the deep cerebellar nuclei?

A. Anterior inferior cerebellar artery
B. Posterior inferior cerebellar artery
C. Superior cerebellar artery
D. Posterior cerebral artery

52.

Within the midbrain, the descending corticospinal tracts are arranged somatotopically. The tracts controlling function of the upper extremity are in which direction compared to tracts controlling the lower extremity?

A. Lateral
B. Posterior
C. Medial
D. Anterior

53.

At the level of the midbrain, fibers conveying sensory information from the upper extremity are in what position relative to the fibers conveying information from the lower extremity?

A. Medial
B. Lateral
C. Anterior
D. Posterior

54.

Which of these structures pass through the tendinous ring of the orbit (annulus of Zinn)?

A. Frontal nerve
B. Trochlear nerve
C. Lacrimal nerve
D. Nasociliary nerve

55.
While exposing the posterior fossa via an extended retrosigmoid craniotomy for a brainstem tumor, you decide to divide the tentorium to increase your superior access. If you inadvertently injure a nerve while dividing the tentorium, what deficit is the patient likely to experience?

A. Lateral rectus palsy
B. Medial rectus palsy
C. Superior oblique palsy
D. Monocular visual loss

56.
You are evaluating a patient for brain death and choose to perform a cold calorics test in the right ear. If the vestibular nuclei are intact, what eye movements do you expect to observe?

A. Nystagmus to the right
B. Nystagmus to the left
C. Superior nystagmus
D. Ocular bobbing

57.
The cochlea is arranged tonotopically. Where are high frequency sounds processed?

A. Base
B. Apex
C. Scala vestibuli
D. Scala tympani

58.
What is the name of the structure that deflects the ciliary processes of the inner and outer hair cells within the cochlea?

A. Tectorial membrane
B. Basilar membrane
C. Scala vestibuli
D. Scala tympani

59.
As a part of the slow acting auditory system, the trapezoid body connects which two structures?

A. Ventral cochlear nucleus–inferior colliculus
B. Ventral cochlear nucleus–medial geniculate body
C. Ventral cochlear nucleus–superior olive
D. Ventral cochlear nucleus–inferior olive

60.
You are watching a 100-m dash at a local track event. You are frightened by the sound of the starting gun and you jump. This response is mediated by the fast-acting auditory pathway. As a part of the fast-acting auditory pathway, the dorsal cochlear nucleus sends fibers to the inferior colliculus via what structure?

A. Medial lemniscus
B. Trapezoid body
C. Lateral lemniscus
D. Restiform body

61.
While evaluating a patient for brain death, you use a small amount of irrigation to the cornea to look for a blink. What brainstem structure mediates this reflex?

A. Spinal trigeminal nucleus
B. Oculomotor nucleus
C. Superior olive
D. Abducens nucleus

62.
Which fibers travel around the abducens nucleus?

A. Spinal trigeminal tract
B. Facial nerve
C. Medial longitudinal fasciculus
D. Internal arcuate fibers

63.
Which hypothalamic nucleus controls satiety?

A. Lateral
B. Ventromedial
C. Paraventricular
D. Preoptic

64.
Which hypothalamic nucleus is involved in fluid balance?

A. Lateral
B. Ventromedial
C. Arcuate
D. Supraoptic

65.
Fibers carrying gustatory information from cranial nerves VII, IX, and X travel between the nucleus of the solitary tract and VPM thalamus via which structure?

A. Central tegmental tract
B. Lateral lemniscus
C. Medial lemniscus
D. Trapezoid body

66.
In order to protect the auditory organs against sudden loud noises, the stapedius and tensor tympani contract to dampen sounds. Which nucleus controls this reflex?

A. Inferior colliculus
B. Superior colliculus
C. Superior olivary nucleus
D. Inferior olivary nucleus

67.
The cribiform plate is part of which cranial bone?

A. Frontal bone
B. Ethmoid bone
C. Zygomatic bone
D. Nasal bone

68.
Which nerve does not pass through the superior orbital fissure?

A. Frontal nerve
B. Maxillary nerve
C. Trochlear nerve
D. Abducens nerve

69.
The vagus nerve exits the base of the skull through what structure?

A. Pars nervosa of the jugular foramen
B. Pars vascularis of the jugular foramen
C. Foramen lacerum
D. Foramen ovale

70.
You are watching a local slow-pitch softball game and someone is hit in the side of the head with a throw at high velocity. As a neurosurgeon, you are worried about the formation of an epidural hematoma. Through what foramen does the main offending artery enter the skull?

A. Foramen ovale
B. Foramen rotundum
C. Foramen spinosum
D. Foramen lacerum

71.
The anterior and posterior ethmoidal arteries are branches from which artery?

A. Carotid artery
B. Internal maxillary artery
C. Sphenopalatine artery
D. Ophthalmic artery

72.
During an endoscopic approach to a pituitary tumor, the middle turbinate is removed by the access surgeon. What is the source of blood supply to the middle turbinate?

A. Anterior ethmoid artery
B. Posterior ethmoid artery
C. Kesselbach's plexus
D. Sphenopalatine artery

73.
What structure separates the optic canal from the superior orbital fissure?

A. Optic strut
B. Anterior clinoid process
C. Carotid process
D. Lateral opticocarotid recess

74.
What is the name of the structure located anterosuperior to the sella turcica, but posterior to the ethmoid air cells?

A. Optic strut
B. Planum sphenoidale
C. Anterior clinoid process
D. Pterygoid plate

75.
The vidian nerve is continuous with which other nerve of the skull base?

A. Lesser superficial petrosal nerve
B. Greater superficial petrosal nerve
C. Nervus intermedius
D. Chorda tympani

76.
Which foramen is just lateral to the vidian canal?

A. Optic canal
B. Foramen rotundum
C. Foramen ovale
D. Foramen spinosum

77.
Which nerve does not run in the double layer of dura making up the lateral wall of the cavernous sinus?

A. Oculomotor nerve
B. Trochlear nerve
C. Ophthalmic nerve
D. Abducens nerve

78.
Which triangle of the skull base is bordered by the inferior aspect of the mandibular nerve, the greater superficial petrosal nerve, and a line drawn between the foramen spinosum and the arcuate eminence?

A.   Glasscock's triangle
B.   Kawase's traingle
C.   Infratrochlear triangle
D.   Trigeminal triangle

79.
Which triangle of the skull base is located superior to the greater superficial petrosal nerve, posterior to the mandibular nerve and anterior to the superior petrosal sinus?

A.   Glasscock's triangle
B.   Kawase's traingle
C.   Infratrochlear triangle
D.   Trigeminal triangle

80.
Which triangle of the skull base is bordered by CN IV, CN V1, and the tentorial edge?

A.   Glasscock's triangle
B.   Kawase's traingle
C.   Infratrochlear triangle
D.   Trigeminal triangle

81.
Bill's bar is a structure within the IAC. Which nerves does it separate?

A.   Facial nerve–cochlear nerve
B.   Superior vestibular nerve–inferior vestibular nerve
C.   Facial nerve–superior vestibular nerve
D.   Cochlear nerve–inferior vestibular nerve

82.
The abducens, facial, and vestibular nerves are associated with which blood vessel in the posterior fossa?

A.   Posterior cerebral artery
B.   Superior cerebellar artery
C.   Anterior inferior cerebellar artery
D.   Posterior inferior cerebellar artery

83.
Which skull landmark is a rough marker of the location of the transverse-sigmoid sinus junction?

A.   Bregma
B.   Inion
C.   Pterion
D.   Asterion

84.
Which is the only cranial nerve to exit on the dorsal aspect of the brainstem?

A.   Oculomotor
B.   Trochlear
C.   Vagus
D.   Hypoglossal

85.
The meninges of the skull base arise from which embryological layer?

A.   Ectoderm
B.   Mesoderm
C.   Endoderm
D.   Somites

86.
Which artery travels with cranial nerves VII and VIII in the IAC?

A.   Posterior inferior cerebellar artery
B.   Calcarine artery
C.   Splenial artery
D.   Labyrinthine artery

87.
What is the first intradural branch of the internal carotid artery?

A.   Meningohypophyseal trunk
B.   Ophthalmic artery
C.   Superior hypophyseal artery
D.   Posterior communicating artery

88.
Special visceral afferent fibers from which cranial nerve do not synapse within the thalamus?

A.   Facial nerve
B.   Hypoglossal nerve
C.   Olfactory nerve
D.   Trigeminal nerve

89.
Axons of which retinal cells make up the optic nerve?

A.   Ganglion cells
B.   Bipolar cells
C.   Horizontal cells
D.   Amacrine cells

90.
Which muscle is not innervated by the inferior division of the oculomotor nerve?

A. Levator palpebrae
B. Inferior oblique
C. Medial rectus
D. Inferior rectus

91.
You are evaluating a patient with a superior oblique palsy, and she leans her head to the left side to compensate for her injury. If the superior oblique palsy is due to damage within the brainstem, which nucleus is involved?

A. Left oculomotor nucleus
B. Right oculomotor nucleus
C. Left trochlear nucleus
D. Right trochlear nucleus

92.
Which cranial nerve mediates the efferent component of the auditory reflex via the tensor tympani?

A. Trigeminal nerve
B. Facial nerve
C. Vestibulocohclear nerve
D. Vagus nerve

93.
You are evaluating a patient who has a lateral gaze palsy of the right eye. During your exam you also notice that the patient cannot cross midline with the left eye on attempted right lateral gaze. Where is the lesion?

A. Left oculomotor nerve
B. Left oculomotor nucleus
C. Right abducens nerve
D. Right abducens nucleus

94.
The nervus intermedius carries fibers for all of the following except?

A. Efferent arm of the corneal reflex
B. Parasympathetic efferents to the lacrimal gland
C. Parasympathetic efferents to the submandibular gland
D. Taste from the anterior two-thirds of the tongue

95.
The cochlear nerve connects which ganglion to which nucleus?

A. Spiral–vestibular nuclei
B. Spiral–cochlear
C. Scarpa's–cochlear
D. Scarpa's–vestibular nuclei

96.
The glossopharyngeal nerve mediates salivation from the parotid gland via which nerve?

A. Lesser superficial petrosal nerve
B. Greater superficial petrosal nerve
C. Vidian nerve
D. Chorda tympani

97.
Which muscle is not innervated by the recurrent branch of the laryngeal nerve?

A. Transverse arytenoid
B. Thyroepiglottic
C. Posterior cricoarytenoid
D. Cricothyroid

98.
The spinal portion of the spinal accessory nerve passes in what location relative to the dentate ligament?

A. Anterior
B. Medial
C. Posterior
D. Lateral

99.
Which extrinsic muscle of the tongue is not innervated by the hypoglossal nerve?

A. Palatoglossus
B. Styloglossus
C. Genioglossus
D. Hyoglossus

100.
The motor root of the trigeminal nerve arises where in relation to the main sensory root of the trigeminal nerve?

A. Caudal
B. Posterior
C. Lateral
D. Rostral

4 Neurobiology

1.
You are caring for an outpatient who has a history of spinal cord injury. You have prescribed oxybutynin for frequent urination. What class of medication is oxybutynin?

A. Muscarinic
B. Anticholinergic
C. Cholinergic
D. Nicotinic
E. Glutamatergic

2.
Astrocytes of the brain sequester what ion?

A. Sodium
B. Potassium
C. Calcium
D. Chloride
E. Magnesium

3.
What receptor utilizes an excitatory neurotransmitter of the brain as a ligand?

A. GABA
B. Ryanodine
C. NMDA
D. Muscarinic
E. Nicotinic

4.
Which of the following hypothalamic nuclei are associated with ADH secretion?

A. Periventricular
B. Lateral
C. Ventromedial
D. Median eminence
E. Supraoptic

5.
Which of the following hypothalamic nuclei is associated with ADH secretion and has diffuse connections in the spinal cord and brainstem?

A. Periventricular
B. Paraventricular
C. Supraoptic
D. Posterior
E. Suprachiasmatic

6.
The use of variable angle screws on a plate during anterior cervical discectomy and fusion surgery helps to diminish what according to Wolf's law?

A. Graft subsidence
B. Screw pullout
C. Development of kyphosis
D. Stress shielding
E. Dysphagia

7.
Activated rhodopsin is involved in phototransduction. What downstream effect does activated rhodopsin have?

A. cGMP deactivation, hyperpolarization
B. cGMP activation, depolarization
C. Potassium channel activation, depolarization
D. Potassium channel activation, hyperpolarization
E. Sodium channel activation, depolarization

8.
Which cortical layer primarily projects back to the thalamus?

A. Layer II
B. Layer III
C. Layer IV
D. Layer V
E. Layer VI

9.
The Betz cells of the cerebral cortex are located in what layer?

A. External pyramidal
B. External granular
C. Multiform
D. Internal pyramidal
E. Internal granular

10.

You decide that on your weekend off you would like to build a supercapacitor in your garage, and you need a phase transfer catalyst to make this system work. You choose TEA, tetraethylammonium, as your agent. During the process, you spill it on the floor and inhale large amounts of the fumes. You start to have difficulty breathing and are slowly becoming paralyzed due to the competitive inhibition of acetylcholine receptors. This compound also affects voltage gated receptors in nerve tissue that are associated with what ion?

A. Sodium
B. Potassium
C. Magnesium
D. Chloride

11.

Myelination of peripheral nerves leads to what?

A. Increased transmembrane resistance, decreased capacitance
B. Increased transmembrane resistance, increased capacitance
C. Decreased transmembrane resistance, increased capacitance
D. Decreased transmembrane resistance, decreased capacitance

12.

A mutation of the gene PTEN is most likely to be seen in the genotyping of what tumor type listed below?

A. Pilocytic astrocytoma
B. WHO grade II glioma
C. Primary GBM
D. Secondary GBM
E. Central neurocytoma

13.

Cerebellar mossy fibers synapse in what region?

A. Granular layer
B. Molecular layer
C. Purkinje layer
D. Multiform layer
E. Pyramidal layer

14.

The Schaffer collateral pathway connects what two regions of the hippocampus?

A. Dentate gyrus–CA1
B. CA1–CA3
C. CA3–subiculum
D. CA1–subiculum
E. Dentate gyrus–subiculum

15.

The perforant pathway of the hippocampus connects what two intrinsic hippocampal structures?

A. Dentate gyrus–CA1
B. CA1–CA3
C. Entorhinal cortex–dentate gyrus
D. CA3–fornix
E. Dentate gyrus–CA1

16.

What receptor type is stimulated by neurons that originate in the substantia nigra pars compacta?

A. Glutamate
B. GABA
C. Dopamine
D. Acetylcholine
E. NMDA

17.

Cortical projections to the striatum use what neurotransmitter?

A. Glutamate
B. GABA
C. Dopamine
D. Acetylcholine
E. Glycine

18.

How many cortical layers are present in the hippocampus?

A. 2
B. 3
C. 4
D. 5
E. 6

19.
You are asked to evaluate a patient with an interesting endocrinologic phenomenon. Her body temperature varies with the temperature of her surrounding environment. She most likely has bilateral destruction of what hypothalamic nucleus?

A.   Anterior nucleus
B.   Posterior nucleus
C.   Ventromedial nucleus
D.   Supraoptic nucleus
E.   Suprachiasmatic nucleus

20.
Destruction of the ventromedial nucleus of the thalamus results in what clinical condition?

A.   Hyperthermia
B.   Anorexia
C.   Hyperphagia
D.   Diabetes insipidus
E.   Addison's disease

21.
Which of the following hypothalamic nuclei is involved with parasympathetic functions?

A.   Anterior nucleus
B.   Posterior nucleus
C.   Lateral nuclei
D.   Ventromedial nucleus
E.   Supraoptic nucleus

22.
You are asked by nursing to evaluate a severely agitated and delirious postoperative patient. He is swinging at nursing and very confused. You decide to give a dose of a medication in the butyrophenone class to treat his agitation. This medication works on what subtype of receptors located in the frontal lobe, the hippocampus, and limbic system.

A.   GABA
B.   Glutamate
C.   Serotonin
D.   D1
E.   D2

23.
You are seeing a patient with severe, unilateral mydriasis. You suspect that the first-order efferent nerve in this pathway is disrupted. What two structures are connected by the first order neuron in this pathway?

A.   Pretectal nucleus – ciliary ganglion
B.   Sympathetic chain – ciliary ganglion
C.   Hypothalamus – sympathetic chain
D.   Hypothalamus – intermediolateral cell column
E.   Ciliary ganglion – radial fibers

24.
You are evaluating a patient in the emergency department with altered mental status, lactic acidosis, and seizures. You suspect cyanide toxicity. What effect does cyanide have on the body?

A.   Blocks voltage-gated potassium channel
B.   Blocks alpha subunit of acetylcholine receptor
C.   Uncouples oxidative phosphorylation
D.   Cleaves synaptobrevin
E.   Inhibits glycine release in the spinal cord

25.
The dorsal motor nucleus of the vagus nerve innervates what target organ(s)?

A.   Muscles of the larynx and pharynx
B.   Thoracic and abdominal viscera
C.   Pharyngeal mucosa
D.   Aortic arch
E.   External ear

26.
Cyclic adenosine monophosphate is a second messenger system for what class of receptors?

A.   Tyrosine kinase
B.   Gprotein
C.   NMDA
D.   Ionotropic

27.
You are working at a neurosurgical clinic in an underdeveloped country. You overhear another physician discussing her patient who drank contaminated water and now has severe diarrhea. The organism has been identified as a vibrio species. You try to remember your basic science days. What receptor protein does the toxin produced by this microbe activate?

A. G_i
B. G_s
C.   cAMP
D. IP_3

28.
Lithium selectively inhibits the phosphatases that degrade what second messenger?

A. DAG
B. Phospholipase C
C. Protein kinase C
D. IP$_3$

29.
Nitric oxide (NO) is liberated after stimulation of what receptor system?

A. Tyrosine kinase
B. G protein
C. NMDA
D. Ionotropic

30.
What ligand would bind to a tyrosine kinase receptor mechanism?

A. Epidermal growth factor
B. Glutamate
C. Benzodiazepine
D. Substance P

31.
Within an acetylcholine-activated receptor system, what specific subunit binds acetylcholine?

A. Alpha
B. Beta
C. Gamma
D. Delta
E. Lambda

32.
You are hiking through Bryce Canyon National Park on your day off and while you are enjoying the beautiful views, you feel a sharp pain in your ankle. You have been bitten by an odd-looking snake that contains alpha-bungarotoxin in its venom. You remember studying this toxin in medical school while you are losing consciousness. What downstream cellular effect is inhibited by alpha-bungarotoxin?

A. Phosphorylation of serine and threonine residues
B. Sodium influx into the cytosol
C. Synthesis of NO
D. Liberation of arachidonic acid from the plasma membrane

33.
Which of these agents is a depolarizing neuromuscular blocker?

A. Vecuronium
B. D-tubocurarine
C. Succinylcholine
D. Gallamine

34.
G-protein coupled muscarinic receptors are located in what CNS location?

A. Dorsal nucleus of Clarke
B. Onuf's nucleus
C. Renshaw cells of the spinal cord
D. Lateral geniculate nucleus

35.
You are called by the emergency department to evaluate a 34-year-old man with new-onset confusion, high fever, and severe spasticity. You discover after looking at X-rays that he has an intrathecal pump in place. You believe the pump is malfunctioning and he is withdrawing from his medication. What receptor does this medication bind to?

A. Muscarinic
B. NMDA
C. GABA$_A$
D. GABA$_B$

36.
What protein stimulates ACh receptor gene transcription in the muscle fiber ultimately leading to increased concentration of ACh receptors in the NMJ?

A. Rapsyn
B. Agrin
C. Neuregulin
D. Muscle-specific tyrosine kinase

37.
Increased calcium concentration within the muscle cell is mediated by what cellular structure?

A. Sarcoplasmic reticulum
B. Endoplasmic reticulum
C. Mitochondria
D. Golgi complex

38.
Sarcomeres are connected to one another by what structure?

A. A band
B. H zone
C. Z disk
D. M line

39.
Which area of the sarcomere shortens during muscle contraction?

A. A band
B. H zone
C. Z disk
D. M line

40.
Ca^{2+} binds with what structure to disinhibit actin binding sites, ultimately allowing actin-myosin crossbridges to be made and muscle contraction to occur?

A. Tropomyosin
B. Troponin I
C. Troponin C
D. Troponin T

41.
You are evaluating a 40-year-old man who is noticing decreased peripheral vision bilaterally. Visual fields demonstrate bitemporal hemianopia. You appropriately order an MRI (demonstrated below). You obtain blood work and discover the following hormone levels

8 AM cortisol = 12 µg/100 mL

Prolactin = 117 ng/mL

IGF-1 = 187 ng/mL

What is the most likely diagnosis?

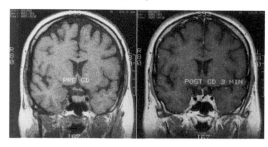

A. Prolactinoma
B. Nonfunctioning pituitary adenoma
C. ACTH-producing adenoma
D. GH-producing adenoma

42.
You resected a difficult suprasellar craniopharyngioma. That evening, the nurse pages you because the patient has had very high urine output for several hours in a row. You order a urine specific gravity, and it returns at 1.003. The depleted hormone you are worried about is released from what structure?

A. Pineal gland
B. Organ vasculosum of the lamina terminalis
C. Adenohypophysis
D. Neurohypophysis

43.
You evaluated a patient in the office with a pituitary mass. She is set to undergo transsphenoidal resection. If her pituitary function tests are listed below, what medication should you give in the postoperative period to avoid complications?

8 AM cortisol = 19 µg/100 mL

Prolactin = 16 ng/mL

IGF-1 = 134 ng/mL

A. Bromocriptine
B. Octreotide
C. DDAVP
D. Hydrocortisone

44.
You have resected a pituitary tumor from a patient with these pituitary function tests preoperatively. What lab test should you order on posterative day 1 to determine the success of the procedure?

8 AM cortisol = 9 µg/100 mL

Prolactin = 22 ng/mL

IGF-1 = 500 ng/mL

A. 8 AM cortisol
B. Sodium
C. Growth hormone
D. IFG-1

45.
Which result below distinguishes a patient as having Cushing's disease versus ectopic ACTH secretion?

A. Random ACTH = 3.4 ng/L
B. 50% reduction in cortisol levels after high dose DMZ suppression test
C. Negative inferior petrosal sinus sampling
D. Negative metyrapone test

46.
What protein is utilized during retrograde axonal transport?

A. Dynamin
B. Dynein
C. Actin/myosin
D. Kinesin

47.
What protein is utilized during fast anterograde axonal transport?

A. Dynamin
B. Dynein
C. Actin/myosin
D. Kinesin

48.
What drug listed below inhibits fast anterograde axonal transport?

A. Temozolomide
B. Carmustine
C. Vinblastine
D. Cyclophosphamide

49.
What is the only neurotransmitter synthesized within the synaptic vesicle?

A. Acetylcholine
B. Norepinephrine
C. Dopamine
D. Glutamate

50.
What is the rate-limiting step for norepinephrine synthesis?

A. Dopamine hydroxylase
B. Aromatic amino acid decarboxylase
C. Tyrosine hydroxylase
D. Choline acetyltransferase

5 Neuropathology

1.

You are evaluating a 65-year-old woman with the onset of low-grade headache and occasional word finding difficulties. Imaging demonstrates a left-sided ring-enhancing mass. You complete a gross total resection and the final pathology is demonstrated below. What gene amplification is often seen in this tumor type?

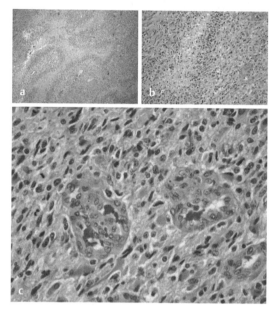

A. VEGF upregulation
B. EGFR amplification
C. 10p/19Q co-deletion
D. SHH deletion

2.

A 30-year-old man experiences a first time seizure after a night of drinking with friends. In the emergency department, a head CT is obtained which is suggestive of a right anterior temporal hypodensity. Subsequent MRI confirms a non-enhancing, T2 hyperintense mass. Surgical resection is performed and final pathology is below. What is the most common chromosomal abnormality in this tumor type?

Use the following figure to answer questions 2 and 3:

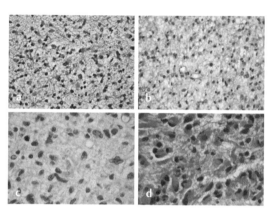

A. Loss of 1P/19Q
B. EGFR amplification
C. Loss of sex chromosome
D. Loss of chromosome 22

3.

You resect a tumor from a 53-year-old man. Final pathology slide is shown in Question 2. What is likely to be demonstrated on further staining of the pathologic tissue?

A. IDH wild-type
B. IDH mutant
C. Loss of chromosome 22
D. Loss of chromosome 10

4.

You see a patient with this MRI. What histologic findings would you expect if this was found to be a glial neoplasm?

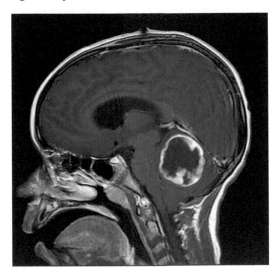

A. Prominent Rosenthal fibers
B. Focal calcification
C. Prominent reticulin staining
D. "Fried-egg appearance"

5.

A 21-year-old woman patient with the tumor demonstrated on this slide is most likely to present with what symptoms?

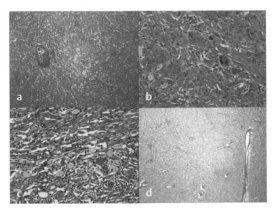

A. Focal neurologic deficit
B. Headache
C. Seizures
D. Nausea

6.

A 30-year-old man patient with the tumor demonstrated on this slide likely has what other abnormalities?

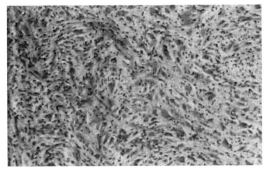

A. Cortical malformations
B. Optic glioma
C. Retinoblastoma
D. Hypotelorism

7.

The tumor seen in this pathology slide often exhibits what genetic abnormality?

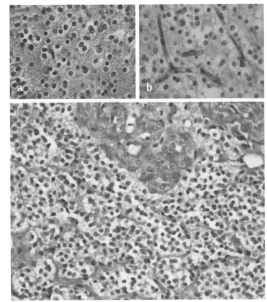

A. Chromosome 17 loss
B. Chromosome 21 loss
C. Isochromosome 17q
D. 1p/19q co-deletion

8.

You resect a tumor in a 40-year-old man that was causing triventricular hydrocephalus. Final pathology is demonstrated below. What characteristic is classic for these tumors?

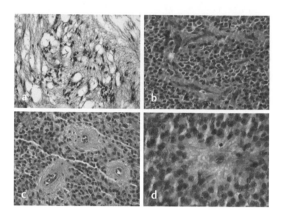

A. S-100 positivity
B. EMA positivity
C. Synaptophysin positivity
D. 1p/19q co-deletion

9.

You resect a tumor in a 60-year-old man that was causing triventricular hydrocephalus. Final pathology is demonstrated below. What characteristic is classic for these tumors?

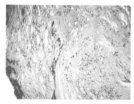
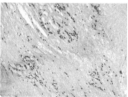

A. Homogenous gadolinium enhancement on MRI
B. Cystic cavity with enhancing mural nodule on MRI
C. Multicentric calcification on CT scan
D. Lack of gadolinium enhancement on MRI

10.

You resect a tumor in a 5-year-old girl with persistent seizures and an abnormality of the temporal lobe on MRI. Final pathology is below. What tumor type did you resect?

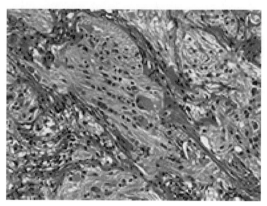

A. Plemorphic xanthoastrocytoma
B. Low-grade glioma
C. Juvenile pilocytic astrocytoma
D. Ganglioglioma

11.

You resect a tumor in a 30-year-old girl. Final pathology is below. This tumor type is often seen in what location?

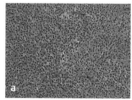
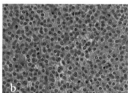

A. Attached to septum pellucidum
B. 4th ventricle
C. Lateral ventricle
D. Temporal lobe

12.
You biopsy a multifocal lesion in the brain of a 60-year-old woman. The final pathology slide is shown below. What is the primary method of initial treatment for this neoplasm?

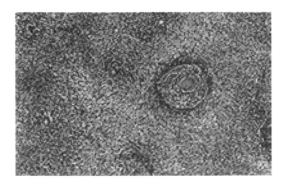

A. Temozolamide/External beam radiotherapy
B. Steroids
C. PCV chemotherapy
D. Stereotactic radiosurgery

13.
The tumor depicted in the slide below originates from which cells?

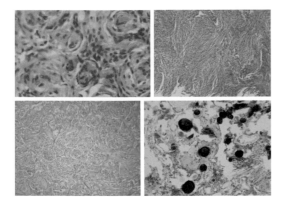

A. Astrocytes
B. Ependymal cells
C. Schwann cells
D. Arachnoid cap cells

14.
What type of meningioma is depicted below?

Use the following figure to answer Questions 14 and 15:

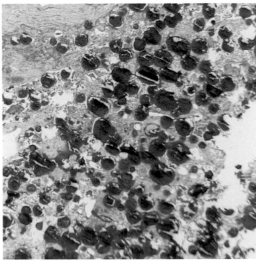

A. Fibrous
B. Psammomatous
C. Transitional
D. Angiomatous

15.
What is the most common genetic malformation in the tumor type depicted in the figure in Question 14?

A. 1p/19q co-deletion
B. Loss of chromosome 22
C. EGFR amplification
D. P53 mutation

16.
Which type of meningioma is considered a WHO grade III lesion?

A. Angiomatous
B. Psammomatous
C. Rhabdoid
D. Chordoid

17.
Meningiomas tend to demonstrate what characteristic positivity?

A. Vimentin
B. GFAP
C. Synaptophysin
D. Neurofilament

18.

A tumor with the histology demonstrated below is most likely to arise from what region?

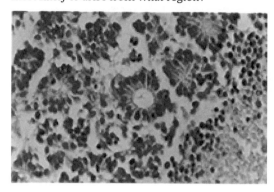

A. Sellar/suprasellar
B. Cerebellum
C. Convexity
D. Pineal

19.

You are evaluating a 52-year-old patient with large hands, coarse fascies, excessive sweating and muscle pain. Ultimately a tumor is resected and the pathology is below. 40% of these tumors exhibit mutations in what gene?

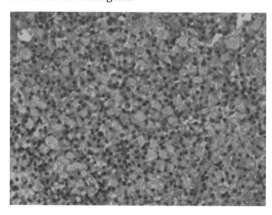

A. n-Myc
B. gsp
C. P53
D. SHH

20.

You are evaluating a patient who is found on imaging to have a large pituitary mass. Pituitary function testing returns normal. You are concerned given the size that pituitary failure will develop. What is the first peptide deficiency you should expect to see?

A. GH
B. FSH/LH
C. TSH
D. ACTH

21.

You resect a mass that appears to be originating in the suprasellar region. Final pathology is demonstrated below. What is the diagnosis?

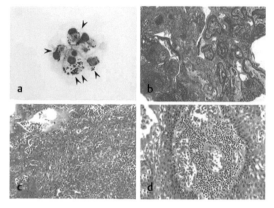

A. Rathke's cleft cyst
B. Germinoma
C. Papillary cranyiopharyngioma
D. Pilocytic astrocytoma

22.

This mass is resected over the convexity, and the final pathology is demonstrated below. What markers distinguish it from a meningioma?

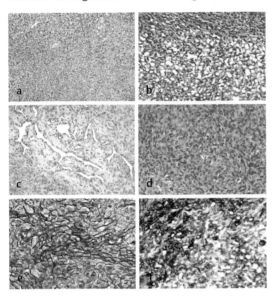

A. EMA positive
B. EMA negative
C. Vimentin positive
D. Vimentin negative

23.

A 42-year-old woman has chronic headaches and undergoes surgery to resect a mass lesion. Final pathology is below. What is the diagnosis?

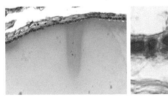

A. Colloid cyst
B. Mature teratoma
C. Pilocytic astrocytoma
D. Dermoid cyst

24.

The mass demonstrated in the pathology slide below originates from what structure?

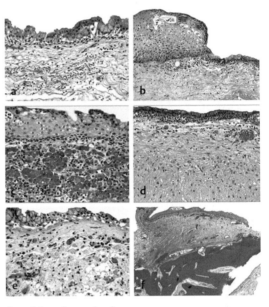

A. Adenohypophysis
B. Pars intermedia
C. Tuburculum sellae
D. Pituitary stalk

25.

A 22-year-old man has this tumor removed after presenting with headaches and nausea. Where is this tumor most likely to arise from?

Use the following figure to answer Questions 25 and 26:

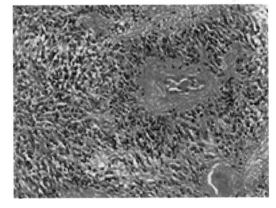

A. Superior medullary velum
B. Floor of the 4th ventricle
C. Choroid plexus
D. C1 nerve root

26.
You would expect the lesion pictured in Question 25 to stain positive for all markers except?

A.   GFAP
B.   Vimentin
C.   EMA
D.   PTAH

27.
You are evaluating a patient who has headaches and received an MRI. The MRI demonstrated a small lesion in the 4th ventricle that does not enhance. The patient is adamant about removing the mass. At surgery, you resect it and send it for pathology, which is demonstrated below. What is the diagnosis?

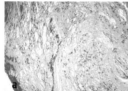

A.   Subependymoma
B.   Ependymoma
C.   Colloid cyst
D.   Schwannoma

28.
If the tumor type below was found to secrete bioactive amines, what is the diagnosis?

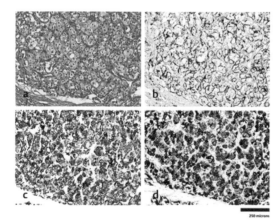

A.   Ganglioglioma
B.   Pleomorphic xanthoastrocytoma
C.   Paraganglioma
D.   Hemangiopericytoma

29.
This MRI demonstrates evidence of what process?

Use the following figure to answer Questions 29 and 30:

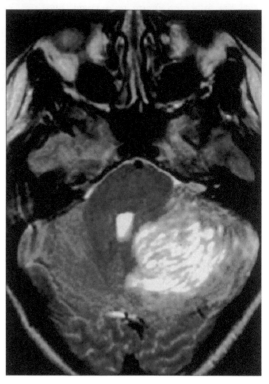

A.   Metastases
B.   Alcoholic cerebellar degeneration
C.   Turcot's syndrome
D.   Lhermitte-Duclos disease

30.
What gene mutation is often linked with patients exhibiting the findings as shown under Question 29?

A.   P53
B.   SHH
C.   PTEN
D.   H-ras

31.
This lesion is resected from the 4th ventricle of a 45-year-old woman. What is the most likely diagnosis?

Use the following figure to answer Questions 31 and 32:

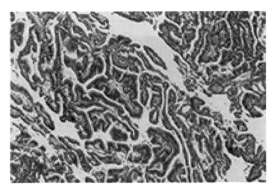

A. Ependymoma
B. Choroid plexus papilloma
C. Subependymoma
D. Vestibular schwannoma

32.
The tumor demonstrated under Question 31 is associated with a syndrome caused by mutation in which gene?

A. P53
B. PTEN
C. SHH
D. H-ras

33.
This tumor is resected from the CP angle of a 55-year-old man. What histologic finding is demonstrated by the black arrow?

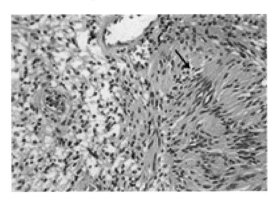

A. Antoni A
B. Antoni B
C. Verocay body
D. Flexner-Wintersteiner rosette

34.
This tumor is resected from the CP angle of a 55-year-old man. What histologic finding is demonstrated in this slide?

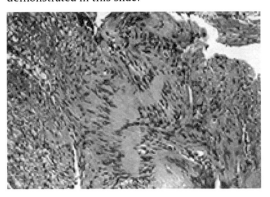

A. Antoni A
B. Antoni B
C. Verocay body
D. Flexner-Wintersteiner rosette

35.
A neurofibroma is thought to arise from what structure?

A. Epineurium
B. Perineurium
C. Endoneurium
D. Schwann cell

36.
A patient with multiple cutaneous nodules has several painful masses resected. They are sent for pathology and are demonstrated below. What is the diagnosis?

Use the following figure to answer Questions 36 and 37:

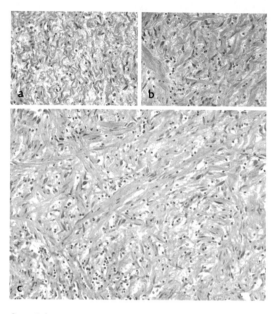

A. Schwannoma
B. Paraganglioma
C. Meningioma
D. Neurofibroma

37.
The lesion depicted in Question 36 most likely stains positive for what marker?

A. S-100
B. CD20
C. Vimentin
D. EMA

38.
A 9-year-old girl presents with wrist drop and a tumor is discovered. The lesion is resected with negative margins and final pathology is demonstrated below. What is the most likely diagnosis?

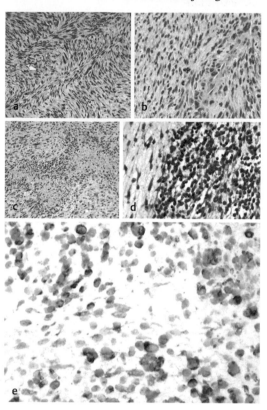

A. Schwannoma
B. MPNST
C. Neuroblastoma
D. Synovial sarcoma

39.
A 42-year-old man has two lesions removed from his cerebellum. Final pathology is below. Mutations on what chromosome are associated with this neoplasm?

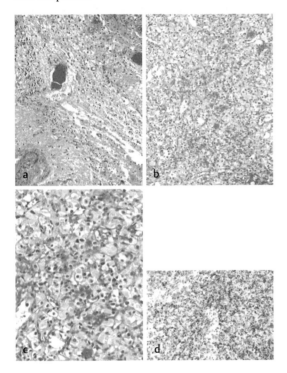

A. 3
B. 7
C. 17
D. 22

40.
This mass is removed from the CP angle in a 28-year-old woman. What is the most likely diagnosis?

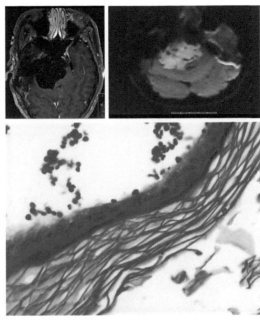

A. Vestibular schwannoma
B. Ependymoma
C. Epidermoid cyst
D. Choroid plexus papilloma

41.
A patient presents to you with tongue deviation to the left and reports that he has been feeling like food is getting stuck in his throat. You resect a mass and the pathology is shown below. What is the most likely diagnosis?

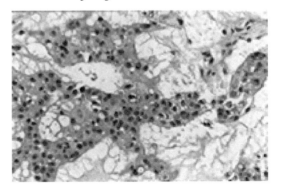

A. Meningioma
B. Ependymoma
C. Epidermoid cyst
D. Chordoma

42.

You resect a mass lesion in a 12-year-old boy with intractable epilepsy. Pre-operative imaging demonstrated an abnormality in the right anterior temporal pole. Final pathology is below, what is the most likely diagnosis?

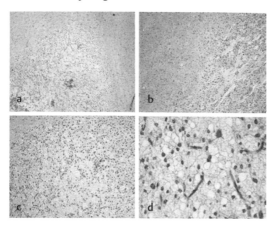

A. PXA
B. Ganglioglioma
C. Dysembryoplastic neuroepithelial tumor
D. Juvenile pilocytic astrocytoma

43.

All of these are subtypes of the tumor depicted below except?

Use the following figure to answer Questions 43, 44 and 49:

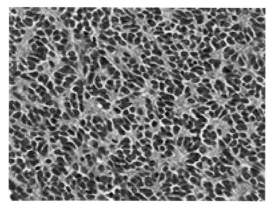

A. Wnt
B. SHH
C. Group 4
D. Group 5

44.

The tumor depicted in Question 43 is thought to arise from what brain region?

A. Floor of the 4th ventricle
B. External granular layer of the cerebellum
C. Choroid plexus
D. Vestibulocochlear nerve

45.

A mass is resected from the suprasellar region in a 14-year-old boy. Final pathology is below. What CSF marker would you expect to be elevated in this patient?

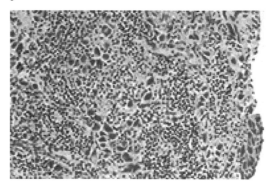

A. Placental alkaline phosphatase
B. B-HCG
C. Glucose
D. Cell count

46.

A mass is resected from the suprasellar region in a 14-year-old boy. Final pathology is below. What CSF marker would you expect to be elevated in this patient?

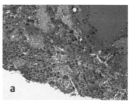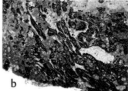

A. Placental alkaline phosphatase
B. B-HCG
C. AFP
D. Cell count

47.
A mass is resected from the suprasellar region in a 14-year-old boy. Final pathology is yolk sac tumor. What CSF marker would you expect to be elevated in this patient?

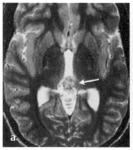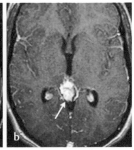

A. Placental alkaline phosphatase
B. B-HCG
C. AFP
D. Cell count

48.
A mass is resected from the suprasellar region in a 14-year-old boy. Final pathology is below. If CSF markers are negative, what is the presumed diagnosis?

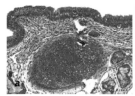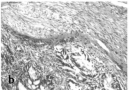

A. Mature teratoma
B. Choriocarcinoma
C. Yolk-sac tumor
D. Medulloblastoma

49.
Of the subtypes of tumor depicted under Question 43, which one has the best prognosis of long-term survival?

A. Wnt
B. SHH
C. Group 3
D. Group 4

50.
This tumor is resected from the midline in a 13-year-old girl, what is the most likely diagnosis?

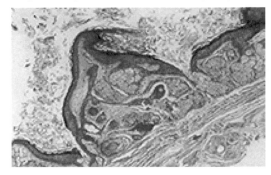

A. Epidermoid cyst
B. Dermoid cyst
C. Germinoma
D. Choriocarcinoma

6 Neuroimaging

1.
A 45-year-old man has an abnormality discovered on MRI. From the MR spectroscopy study shown in the following image, what is the most likely diagnosis?

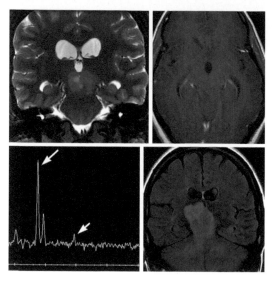

A. Abscess
B. Infarction
C. Glioma
D. Hemorrhage

2.
A 73-year-old man has an abnormality discovered on MRI. The MR spectroscopy study indicates an elevated lactate. What is the most likely diagnosis?

A. Abscess
B. Infarction
C. Glioma
D. Hemorrhage

3.
A 55-year-old man undergoes resection of a right frontal glioblastoma. He undergoes a standard temozolomide and radiation regimen postoperatively. Nine months later, enhancement is seen within the resection cavity. MR spectroscopy demonstrates the NAA peak to be double the choline peak. What is the most likely diagnosis?

A. Abscess
B. Infarction
C. Recurrent glioma
D. Radiation necrosis

4.
This MRI is from a 50-year-old woman who was having headaches. What mutation listed below would suggest that this lesion is primary and not due to malignant transformation?

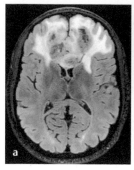
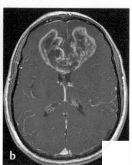

A. PTEN mutant
B. PTEN wild type
C. IDH-1 mutant
D. IDH-1 wild type

5.
What is the most likely diagnosis?

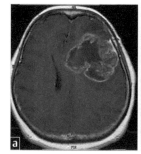
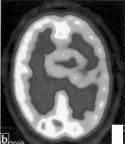

A. Glioblastoma
B. Infarction
C. Hemorrhage
D. Huntington's disease

6.

What is the most likely diagnosis?

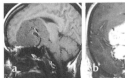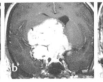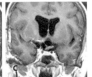

A. Glioblastoma
B. Meningioma
C. Metastasis
D. Low-grade glioma

7.

If final pathology of the image below comes back as chordoid type, what WHO grade is the lesion?

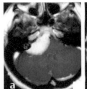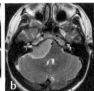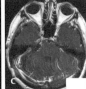

A. WHO grade I
B. WHO grade II
C. WHO grade III
D. WHO grade IV

8.

What is the most likely diagnosis?

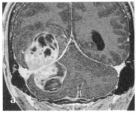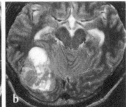

A. Glioblastoma
B. Metastasis
C. Hemangiopericytoma
D. Fibrous dysplasia

9.

Where are the lesions pictured below most often located within the brain?

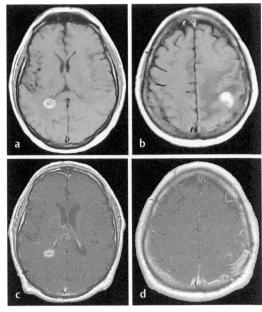

A. Cortical surface
B. Gray–white matter junction
C. White matter
D. Ependymal lining

10.

This MRI demonstrates a metastatic lesion with edema. What is the most likely primary source?

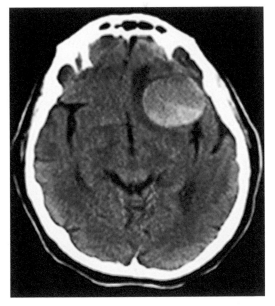

A. Skin
B. Lung
C. Breast
D. Colon

11.
What chromosomal abnormality does the patient with the MRI findings below most likely have?

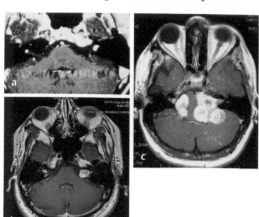

A. 3
B. 7
C. 17
D. 22

12.
What is the most likely diagnosis?

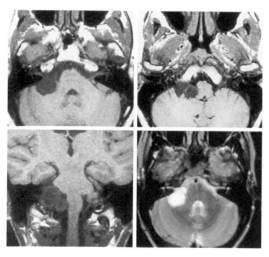

A. Vestibular schwannoma
B. Epidermoid cyst
C. Petrous meningioma
D. Ependymoma

13.
A 45-year-old man presents with headaches and persistent nausea prompting an MRI pictured below. What is the most likely diagnosis?

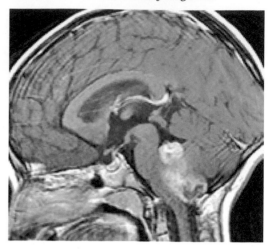

A. Vestibular schwannoma
B. Epidermoid cyst
C. Subependymoma
D. Ependymoma

14.
A 45-year-old man presents with headaches and persistent nausea prompting an MRI pictured below. What foramen is this tumor extending through?

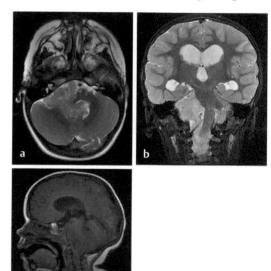

A. Magendie
B. Luschka
C. Magnum
D. Lacerum

15.
A 52 year-old woman presents with persistent headaches prompting an MRI pictured below. What is the most likely diagnosis?

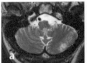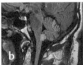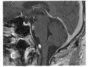

A. Ependymoma
B. Subependymoma
C. Vestibular schwannoma
D. Medulloblastoma

16.
A 52-year-old woman presents with a severe headache that resolves. An MRI is obtained and is shown below. What is the most likely diagnosis?

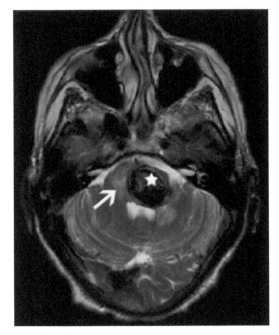

A. Ependymoma
B. Subependymoma
C. Vestibular schwannoma
D. PICA aneurysm

17.
A 28-year-old man has sudden onset of dysarthria and a left sixth nerve palsy. MRI is shown below. What is the most likely diagnosis?

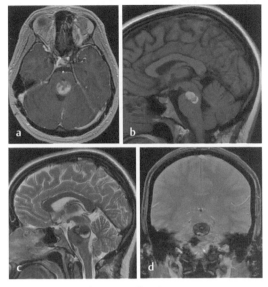

A. Dural arteriovenous fistula
B. Arteriovenous malformation
C. Cavernous malformation
D. Aneurysm

18.
A patient is set to undergo a Wada test to determine language dominance. Before the procedure commences, a standard angiogram is performed. In this lateral DSA of the internal carotid artery, what is demonstrated?

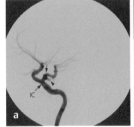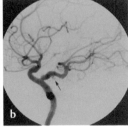

A. PICA aneurysm
B. Dural arteriovenous malformation
C. Fetal posterior cerebral artery
D. Persistent trigeminal artery

19.
A 54-year-old woman has an abnormality discovered on routine MRI and undergoes a formal cerebral angiogram, which is pictured below. What type of aneurysm is this?

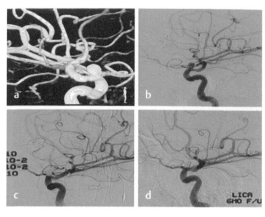

A. Posterior communicating artery aneurysm
B. Carotid-ophthalmic aneurysm
C. Superior hypophyseal aneurysm
D. Cavernous sinus aneurysm

20.
Where is this aneurysm located?

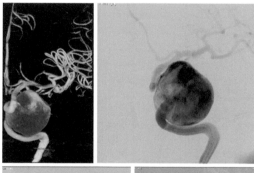
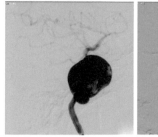
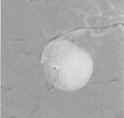

A. Intracranial/intradural
B. Intracranial/extradural
C. Extracranial/intradural
D. Extracranial/extradural

21.
What structure is demonstrated (arrows, not arrowheads) in this angiogram in a patient with a sagittal sinus thrombosis?

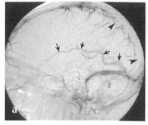
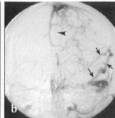

A. Anastomotic vein of Trolard
B. Anastomotic vein of Labbé
C. Vein of Galen
D. Petrosal sinus

22.
What characteristic makes this a pituitary macroadenoma?

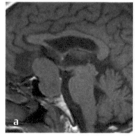
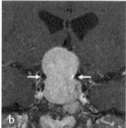

A. Encirclement of the carotid
B. Optic nerve compression
C. Size greater than 10 cm
D. Size greater than 2.0 cm

23.
What is the most likely diagnosis?

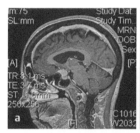
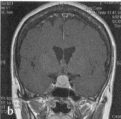

A. Pituitary macroadenoma
B. Craniopharyngioma
C. Tuberculum meningioma
D. Chordoma

24.
An 8-year-old boy is developing slowly progressive visual loss prompting an MRI shown below. What condition is this mass associated with?

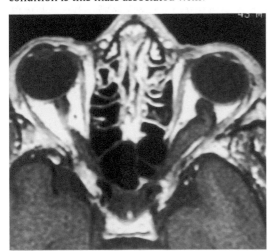

A. NF1
B. NF2
C. Tuberous sclerosis
D. Cowden's syndrome

25.
An 8-year-old boy has headaches and an MRI is performed. The lesion pictured below is associated with a syndrome caused by which chromosomal abnormality?

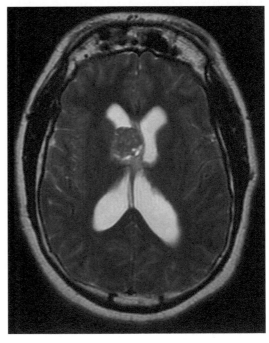

A. 17
B. 22
C. 9
D. 3

26.
What structure does number 8 in this MRI demonstrate?

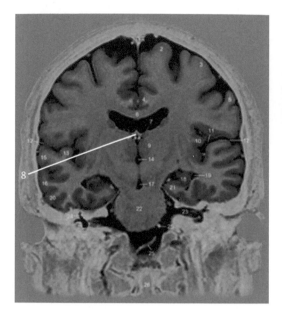

27.
What structure does number 18 in this coronal, T2-weighted MRI demonstrate?

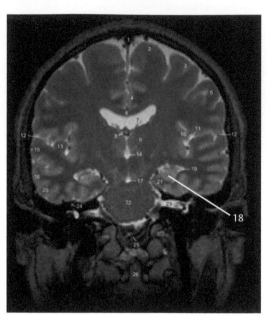

A. Septum pellucidum
B. Basal vein of Rosenthal
C. Choroid plexus
D. Internal cerebral veins

A. Limen insulae
B. Amygdala
C. Diagonal band of Broca
D. Hippocampus

28.
A 65-year-old man has sudden onset of headache and starts having difficulty controlling generalized tonic–clonic seizures in the emergency department. Ultimately, he requires intubation for seizure control. MRI is shown below; what is the most likely diagnosis?

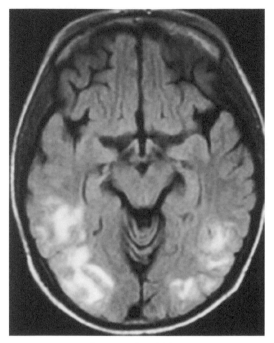

A. Aneurysmal subarachnoid hemorrhage
B. Metastatic tumor
C. Posterior reversible encephalopathy syndrome
D. Multiple system atrophy

29.
A 62-year-old man has sudden onset of headache and starts having difficulty controlling generalized tonic–clonic seizures in the emergency department. Ultimately, he requires intubation for seizure control. MRI is shown below; what is the next best step?

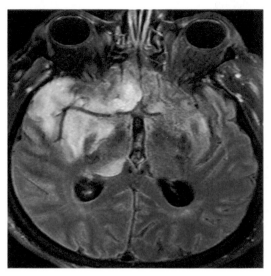

A. Start acyclovir
B. Start barbiturates
C. Check blood sugar
D. Arrange for needle biopsy

30.
You are seeing a 35-year-old man with difficulty controlling seizures. The MRI scan is demonstrated below. What is the most likely diagnosis?

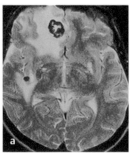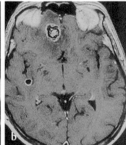

A. Metastases
B. Neurocysticercosis
C. Familial cavernomatosis
D. Gliomatosis cerebri

31.
You are asked to evaluate a 2-month-old infant who has been found to have hydrocephalus and altered mental status. Head CT is demonstrated below. What is the most likely diagnosis?

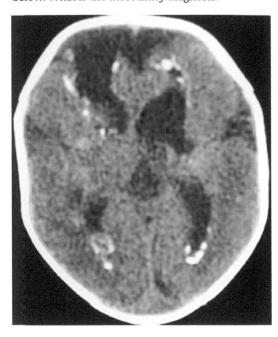

A. Aqueductal stenosis
B. Cytomegalovirus (CMV) encephalitis
C. Germinal matrix hemorrhage
D. Vein of Galen malformation

32.
You are evaluating a 46-year-old woman with a history of headaches and intermittent clumsiness of the left hand that resolves completely several weeks after onset. MRI is demonstrated below. What is the most likely diagnosis?

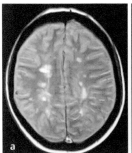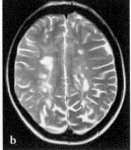

A. Multiple sclerosis
B. CNS lymphoma
C. Metastases
D. Gliomatosis cerebri

33.
You are evaluating a 37-year-old woman with a history of headaches and intermittent neurologic deficits that seem to resolve completely over time. Now she is in the emergency department with a GCS of 12 (E3, V4, M5). MRI is demonstrated below. What is the most likely diagnosis?

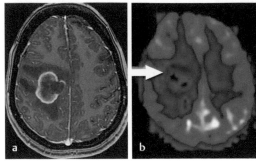

A. Balo's concentric sclerosis
B. CNS lymphoma
C. Tumefactive multiple sclerosis
D. Glioblastoma

34.
The syndrome that causes the findings on this MRI is due to abnormality in what cellular process?

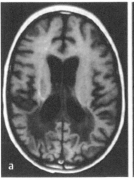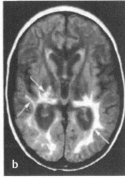

A. Very long chain fatty acid synthesis
B. Glucocerebrosidase deficiency
C. Isocitrate dehydrogenase deficiency
D. Glycogen storage

35.
You are evaluating a 35-year-old homeless man who reports intravenous (IV) drug use who has developed persistent headaches. An abnormality is seen on CT; findings are shown below. What is the most likely diagnosis?

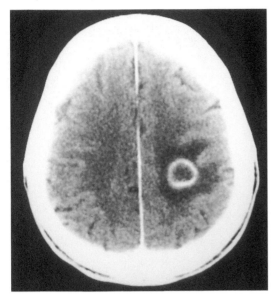

A. Metastasis
B. Cerebral abscess
C. Glioblastoma
D. Meningioma

36.
You are evaluating a 35-year-old homeless man who has developed persistent headaches. An abnormality is seen on CT scan prompting an MRI; findings are shown below. If the diagnosis of a cerebral abscess is confirmed, what would be the most likely isolate?

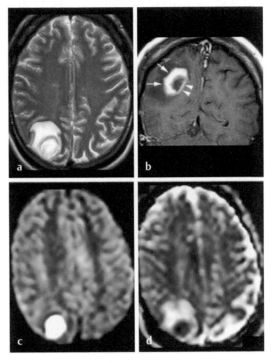

A. *Streptococcus milleri*
B. *Listeria monocytogenes*
C. *Staphylococcus aureus*
D. *Klebsiella pneumoniae*

37.

A 26-year-old woman is 6 months postpartum and is found to be in diabetes insipidus by her primary care provider. An MRI is obtained and is demonstrated below. What is the most likely diagnosis?

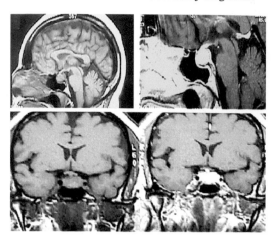

A. Pituitary macroadenoma
B. Craniopharyngioma
C. Pituitary apoplexy
D. Lymphocytic hypophysitis

38.

A 26-year-old woman is 3 days post vaginal delivery that was complicated by uterine hemorrhage resulting in approximately 2 L of blood loss. On postpartum day 3, her blood pressure suddenly increases due to pain while walking and she experiences onset of headaches and visual disturbances. An MRI is demonstrated below. What should be your next step?

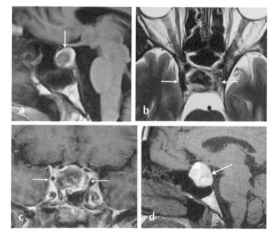

A. Emergent pituitary decompression
B. Obtain MRI
C. Check sodium
D. Give hydrocortisone

39.

A 67-year-old man has onset of right facial droop, tongue deviation to the left, and some dysmetria on finger–nose–finger testing. Postcontrast MRI is demonstrated below. What is the most likely diagnosis?

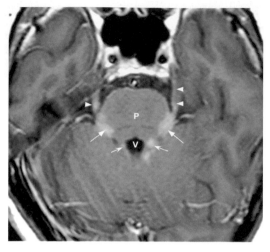

A. CNS lymphoma
B. Leptomeningeal carcinomatosis
C. Neurosarcoidosis
D. Acute disseminated encephalomyelitis

40.

Which neurotransmitter does the structure identified by number 2 in this coronal MRI use?

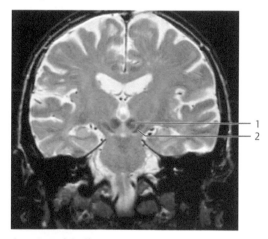

A. Acetylcholine
B. Dopamine
C. Norepinephrine
D. Serotonin

41.
An 80-year-old man has started to develop changes in personality and socially disruptive behavior. More recently, his language has been affected. MRI is demonstrated below. What is the most likely diagnosis?

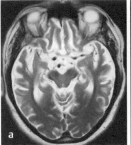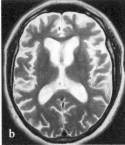

A. Corticobasal degeneration
B. Parkinson's disease
C. Frontotemporal dementia
D. Alzheimer's disease

42.
What signal intensity on T1-weighted imaging does hyperacute (< 24) hemorrhage demonstrate?

A. Isointense
B. Hyperintense
C. Hypointense
D. Hyperdense

43.
What signal intensity on T2-weighted imaging does hyperacute (< 24) hemorrhage demonstrate?

A. Isointense
B. Hyperintense
C. Hypointense
D. Hyperdense

44.
What signal intensity on T2-weighted imaging does acute (1–3 days) hemorrhage demonstrate?

A. Isointense
B. Hyperintense
C. Hypointense
D. Hyperdense

45.
What signal intensity on T1-weighted imaging does acute (1–3 days) hemorrhage demonstrate?

A. Isointense
B. Hyperintense
C. Hypointense
D. Hyperdense

46.
What signal intensity on T1-weighted imaging does early subacute (3–7 days) hemorrhage demonstrate?

A. Isointense
B. Hyperintense
C. Hypointense
D. Hyperdense

47.
What signal intensity on T2-weighted imaging does early subacute (3–7 days) hemorrhage demonstrate?

A. Isointense
B. Hyperintense
C. Hypointense
D. Hyperdense

48.
What signal intensity on T2-weighted imaging does late subacute (7–14 days) hemorrhage demonstrate?

A. Isointense
B. Hyperintense
C. Hypointense
D. Hyperdense

49.
What signal intensity on T1-weighted imaging does late subacute (7–14 days) hemorrhage demonstrate?

A. Isointense
B. Hyperintense
C. Hypointense
D. Hyperdense

50.
What signal intensity on T1-weighted imaging does chronic (> 14 days) hemorrhage demonstrate?

A. Isointense
B. Hyperintense
C. Hypointense
D. Hyperdense

7 Fundamental Skills

1.
Approximately what percentage of total body fluid is intravascular?

A. 3%
B. 8%
C. 25%
D. 50%
E. 75%

2.
You evaluate a patient in the emergency department who has a history of a syringopleural shunt and now is having difficulty breathing. Chest X-ray is shown. What treatment should you consider in this patient?

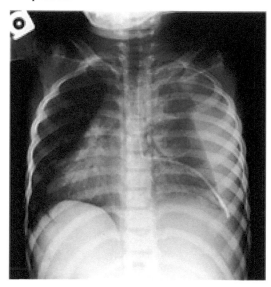

A. Diuretics
B. Needle decompression
C. Shunt externalization/removal
D. Antibiotics
E. Observation

3.
What finding on invasive monitoring would a patient with cardiogenic pulmonary edema likely have?

A. Hypoxemia with a normal A–a gradient
B. PCWP > 18 mm Hg
C. PCWP < 18 mm Hg
D. PAO_2/FiO_2 255 mm Hg
E. Hypoventilation with normal A–a gradient

4.
What medication can be used in patients with severe ARDS to improve oxygenation?

A. Diuretics
B. Dobutamine
C. Dexamethasone
D. Beta blocker
E. Nimodipine

5.
In treating what type of arrhythmia is adenosine useful?

A. Narrow complex tachycardia
B. Wide complex tachycardia
C. Ventricular fibrillation
D. Atrial fibrillation
E. Wolff–Parkinson–White syndrome

6.
You are caring for a patient in the ICU who has suddenly developed a wide complex tachycardia. She is awake, conversive, and currently stable. What would be an appropriate treatment for her condition?

A. Defibrillation
B. Lidocaine infusion
C. Coronary angiogram
D. tPA administration
E. Adenosine

7.
You are evaluating a new admission to the neuro-ICU. The patient was involved in a motor vehicle collision and currently demonstrates flexor posturing of the upper extremities, briefly opens his eyes to pain, and is nonverbal. What is his GCS score?

A. 15
B. 0
C. 3
D. 6
E. 9

8.
In the neuro-ICU, you are called by a nurse to evaluate a patient with pupillary abnormalities. When you see the patient, you observe rhythmic dilation and contraction of the pupillary sphincter muscles. What is causing this?

A. Normal physiologic response
B. Uncal herniation
C. Diabetic oculomotor palsy
D. Transient ischemic attacks
E. Shearing injury of the oculomotor nerve

9.
You are caring for a patient in the neuro-ICU after an intracerebral hemorrhage. She has baseline progressive dementia. In the ICU, her delirium worsens significantly in the evening and at night. This condition is thought to be due to degeneration of what hypothalamic nucleus?

A. Anterior nucleus
B. Ventromedial nucleus
C. Suprachiasmatic nucleus
D. Supraoptic nucleus
E. Lateral nucleus

10.
Which of the following is not a type of opioid receptor?

A. Mu
B. Delta
C. Kappa
D. N/OFQ
E. Gamma

11.
Which of the following coagulation cascade factors is inhibited by warfarin?

A. 3
B. 5
C. 8
D. 9
E. 12

12.
Approximately how long will it take for IV vitamin K to normalize the INR in a patient who is anticoagulated with warfarin?

A. 4 hours
B. 8 hours
C. 12 hours
D. 18 hours
E. 24+ hours

13.
On what coagulation factor does the combination of heparin/antithrombin exert anticoagulant effects?

A. III
B. VII
C. IX
D. Xa
E. XII

14.
You are treating a patient in the ICU who is in acute renal failure and needs to have DVT prophylaxis initiated. Unfortunately, she has developed heparin-induced thrombocytopenia and you need another option. Which of the following anticoagulants would be contraindicated in her current condition?

A. Aspirin
B. Dabigatran
C. Argatroban
D. Warfarin
E. Clopidogrel

15.
What is the approximate half-life of aspirin?

A. 30 minutes
B. 6 hours
C. 24 hours
D. 7 days
E. 1 month

16.
Via what mechanism does clopidogrel exhibit an antiplatelet effect?

A. Inhibition of thromboxane synthesis via COX 1 inhibition
B. $P2Y_{12}$ receptor binding inhibiting ADP mediated platelet aggregation (GPIIb/IIIa)
C. Thienopyridine-mediated ADP receptor blockade
D. Factor IIa inhibition
E. Binds antithrombin III

17.
What level of urine output suggests adequate volume replacement?

A. 0.1 to 0.5 mL/kg/h
B. 0.5 to 1.0 mL/kg/h
C. 1.0 to 1.5 mL/kg/h
D. 1.5 to 2.0 mL/kg/h
E. 2.0 to 2.5 mL/kg/h

18.

What is the best immediate reversal agent of a patient with an elevated INR and ICH who also has coexistent heart failure?

A. Prothrombin complex concentrates
B. Fresh frozen plasma
C. IV vitamin K
D. Transexamic acid
E. Protamine

19.

You are about to discharge a hospitalized patient who is now at POD 3 from a lumbar laminectomy. Her hospital course was complicated by development of an unprovoked left lower extremity DVT. It has been recommended that she discharge on oral anticoagulation for treatment of her DVT. How long should she be on anticoagulation for this event?

A. 1 week
B. 1 month
C. 3 months
D. 6 months
E. 1 year

20.

You are caring for a 33-year-old woman who is on oral contraceptive pills and intermittently smokes. She developed a severe headache and has the findings demonstrated in the images below. What is the best initial management of her condition?

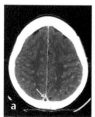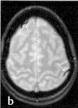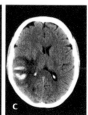

A. Intravenous heparin
B. Observation
C. Aspirin
D. TransarterialtPA
E. Dabigatran administration

21.

What brain tissue partial pressure of oxygen level is thought to be the threshold below which anaerobic respiration takes over and secondary injury via lactic acidosis occurs?

A. 50 mm Hg
B. 40 mm Hg
C. 30 mm Hg
D. 20 mm Hg
E. 10 mm Hg

22.

According to the guidelines for the management of severe traumatic brain injury, a GCS of what is considered severe head injury?

A. 12 or less
B. 10 or less
C. 8 or less
D. 6 or less
E. 3

23.

You are asked to evaluate a patient with a severe head injury in the ED after a motor vehicle collision. As you are arriving to the ED, you see the ED resident starting to intubate. You are told that the patient was given rocuronium for paralytic just prior to intubation. How long will you likely have to wait before you can get an adequate neurologic exam?

A. 15 minutes
B. 30 minutes
C. 90 minutes
D. 6 hours
E. 24 hours

24.

Via what mechanism can hyperventilation of the intubated patient with elevated ICP decrease ICP?

A. Decreased pH
B. Increased pH
C. Increased CSF production
D. Decreased CSF production
E. Decreased cardiac output

25.

You are evaluating a patient who has suffered a severe brain injury and unfortunately no measures have led to improvement of the patient's condition. He is currently on comfort cares and as you observe, his breathing pattern consists of a prolonged pause at full inspiration. Where does this breathing pattern localize the injury?

A. Diffuse forebrain
B. Thalamus
C. Pons
D. Medulla
E. Upper cervical spine

26.

What is the average cerebral blood flow to the brain in the normal, healthy adult?

A. 20 mL/100 g/min
B. 35 mL/100 g/min
C. 50 mL/100 g/min
D. 75 mL/100 g/min
E. 100 mL/100 g/min

27.

What is the normal cerebral blood flow in a normal, healthy 4-year-old?

A. 20 mL/100 g/min
B. 35 mL/100 g/min
C. 50 mL/100 g/min
D. 75 mL/100 g/min
E. 100 mL/100 g/min

28.

Which of the following tumors is associated with hyponatremia?

A. Bronchogenic carcinoma
B. Small cell lung cancer
C. Medullary thyroid cancer
D. Neuroblastoma
E. Medulloblastoma

29.

You are evaluating a 38-year-old woman who has severe migraines, several seizure episodes, and a recent subclinical stroke that was demonstrated on MRI. She also has an associated mood disorder. Dilutional testing is suggestive of an inhibitor present. You suspect lupus. How do you confirm the diagnosis of neuropsychiatric SLE?

A. Skin biopsy
B. CSF antineuronal antibodies
C. CSF anti-Jo antibodies
D. CSF anti-RI antibodies
E. CSF glucose

30.

You are evaluating a 64-year-old woman with left arm and leg weakness. MRI has the following findings. Genetic testing demonstrates an abnormality on chromosome 19. What is the diagnosis?

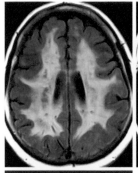
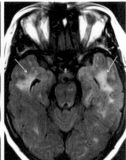
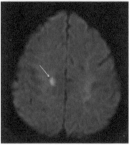

A. Alexander's disease
B. CADASIL
C. PML
D. Symptomatic carotid stenosis
E. Multiple embolic infarcts

31.

You are evaluating a 76-year-old man who presents with persistent temporal headaches, jaw claudication, and tenderness of the temporal artery. If this patient were to go on to develop blindness, what mechanism underlies the ischemic optic neuropathy?

A. Inflammation
B. Thrombosis
C. Embolic infarct
D. Arterial rupture

32.

You are caring for a patient with giant cell arteritis, newly diagnosed. You are concerned about the development of blindness in this patient. What should be your initial management?

A. Clopidogrel
B. Heparin
C. Prednisone
D. Hydroxychloroquine
E. Infliximab

33.

What serum osmolality represents a threshold after which mannitol administration is contraindicated due to an elevated risk of acute tubular necrosis?

A. 300
B. 310
C. 320
D. 330
E. 340

34.

You are asked to review the CT scan of a 7-week-old newborn with a head mass. What is the diagnosis?

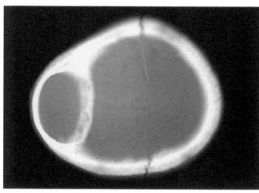

A. Epidermoid cyst
B. Eosinophilic granuloma
C. Growing skull fracture
D. Calcified cephalohematoma
E. Nonaccidental trauma

35.

You are asked to evaluate a 5-day-old newborn who has a cephalohematoma that has not resolved at this point. It does not appear to have increased in size; the child remains afebrile and stable both neurologically and systemically. What treatment should you recommend?

A. Further observation
B. Surgical decompression
C. Needle aspiration
D. Serial CT scans
E. Tight head wrap

36.

Retinal hemorrhages are a classic symptom of severe, abusive pediatric head trauma, occurring in up to 80% of patients. How often are retinal hemorrhages present in cases of confirmed accidental trauma?

A. 5%
B. 15%
C. 35%
D. 55%
E. 75%

37.

You are seeing a patient in the ED. You were called emergently as this patient has evidence of an epidural hematoma and has now developed pupillary anisocoria. You decide to go emergently to the OR for evacuation. Based on current evidence, after the onset of pupillary changes, within what time interval should you achieve decompression of the hematoma to promote a good outcome?

A. < 10 minutes
B. < 70 minutes
C. < 120 minutes
D. < 6 hours
E. < 24 hours

38.

Which of the following measurements of an acute subdural hematoma meets criteria for evacuation regardless of GCS?

A. 7-mm thick/4-mm midline shift
B. 12-mm thick/6-mm midline shift
C. 3-mm thick/3-mm midline shift
D. 9-mm thick/2-mm midline shift
E. 13-mm thick/1-mm midline shift

39.

You are caring for a patient who has developed postsurgical brachial neuritis (Parsonage–Turner syndrome). She is experiencing significant shoulder girdle pain. What medication should you use to help her symptoms?

A. Prednisone
B. NSAIDs
C. Ketamine
D. Methotrexate
E. Temozolomide

40.
In patients with nonhereditary brachial neuritis (Parsonage–Turner syndrome), what is the expected rate of full recovery at 3 years?

A. 50%
B. 60%
C. 70%
D. 90%
E. 100%

41.
Which of the following is a known side effect of dexmedetomidine use for sedation in the neuro-ICU?

A. Seizures
B. Agitation
C. Bradycardia
D. Hypertension
E. Tachycardia

42.
What brainstem nucleus is thought to be mediated by administration of dexmedetomidine?

A. Raphe nucleus
B. Nucleus accumbens
C. Periaqueductalgray
D. Locus coeruleus
E. Solitary tract

43.
Only for what time frame is continuous infusion of dexmedetomidine approved by the FDA?

A. 1 hour
B. 6 hours
C. 12 hours
D. 24 hours
E. 48 hours

44.
What might you see as an initial symptom of propofol infusion syndrome in a patient who has received high doses of propofol for the last 72 hours?

A. Hypertension
B. New right bundle branch block
C. Seizures
D. Metabolic alkalosis
E. Hypokalemia

45.
Which of the following anesthetic agents inhibits the formation of ACTH?

A. Propofol
B. Etomidate
C. Ketamine
D. Pentobarbital
E. Isoflurane

46.
Which of the following conditions would be a contraindication to performing a supracerebellar, infratentorial approach to a pineal region tumor in the sitting position?

A. Patent foramen ovale
B. Pre-existing DVT
C. Restrictive lung disease
D. History of cervical fusion
E. Ongoing cervical radiculopathy

47.
Which of the following anesthetic medications can lower the seizure threshold?

A. Propofol
B. Pentobarbital
C. Etomidate
D. Midazolam
E. Methohexital

48.
You are evaluating a 38-year-old man with right-sided temporal lobe epilepsy from presumed hippocampal sclerosis. According to the landmark controlled trial focusing on temporal lobe epilepsy, what percentage of surgical patients will be completely seizure free at 1 year?

A. ~ 25%
B. ~ 33%
C. ~ 40%
D. ~ 60%
E. ~ 90%

49.
You are evaluating a 52-year-old man with medically refractory epilepsy that appears to be located in eloquent cortex (motor cortex) on the right side. There are no other options and you and the patient are considering a procedure to perform multiple pial transections in attempt to control the epilepsy. What should you council this patient about during the postoperative course?

A. Permanent motor deficit
B. Temporary motor deficit
C. Initial seizure worsening
D. High risk of infection
E. High risk of postoperative hemorrhage

50.
You are seeing a patient in clinic with drug-resistant epilepsy who is being considered for surgical treatment. She describes her seizure onset including a rising epigastric sensation just prior to initiation of her seizure episode. Where is the most likely location of her epilepsy?

A. Medial frontal lobe
B. Occipital lobe
C. Temporal lobe
D. Lateral frontal lobe
E. Parietal lobe

51.
Which of the following factors is more consistent with type II or atypical trigeminal neuralgia?

A. Lancinating pain
B. Pain-free intervals
C. Unilateral
D. Throbbing pain

52.
What percentage of patients with classic type I trigeminal neuralgia pain will have "excellent to good" pain relief long term with microvascular decompression?

A. 25%
B. 65%
C. 75%
D. 85%
E. 95%

53.
What percentage of patients with atypical type II trigeminal neuralgia pain will have "excellent to good" pain relief long term with microvascular decompression?

A. 25%
B. 65%
C. 75%
D. 85%
E. 95%

54.
You are asked to see a patient who is having severe, episodic pain in the right lower jaw. She describes lancinating pain that is worsened by brushing her teeth. You suspect trigeminal neuralgia. What is the best initial management of her condition?

A. Balloon compression
B. Radiofrequency rhizotomy
C. Microvascular decompression
D. Medical management
E. Glycerol rhizotomy

55.
What is the mechanism of action for trigeminal neuralgia pain relief via administration of the medication oxcarbazepine?

A. Voltage-gated sodium channel blockade
B. Voltage-gated calcium channel blockade
C. Mu opioid receptor agonist
D. NMDA receptor agonist
E. GABA agonist

56.
You are performing a balloon compression of the trigeminal nerve in a patient with TN. If the patient has primarily V3 distribution pain, where in the foramen ovale should you attempt to place the catheter?

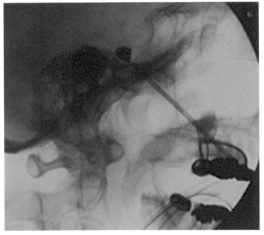

A. Superior
B. Inferior
C. Lateral
D. Medial
E. Intermediate

57.
Which of the following patients is most likely to have the findings on MRI demonstrated below?

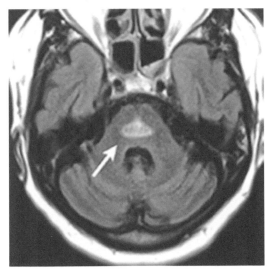

A. A 67-year-old woman with breast cancer
B. A 55-year-old male alcoholic
C. A 42-year-old male IV drug user
D. An 18-year-old woman with lymphoma
E. An 80-year-old woman with carotid stenosis

58.
Which of the following conditions causes peaked T waves on ECG?

A. Hypokalemia
B. Hyperkalemia
C. Hypomagnesemia
D. Hypercalcemia
E. Hypernatremia

59.
You are reading an ECG that demonstrates prolongation of the PR interval. What electrolyte abnormality can cause this finding on ECG?

A. Hyponatremia
B. Hypocalcemia
C. Hyperkalemia
D. Hypernatremia
E. Hypermagnesemia

60.
Hypomagnesemia can lead to what changes on ECG?

A. Prolonged PR interval
B. ST elevation
C. Multifocality
D. QRS prolongation
E. Bundle branch block

61.
Which of the following is a contraindication to the use of IV rtPA in the treatment of acute ischemic stroke?

A. Cortical-based tumor
B. Symptoms for 4 hours
C. History of seizures
D. Age of 18 years
E. Platelet count of 115,000

62.
Occlusion of the PICA proximal to what point will likely result in a lateral medullary syndrome?

A. Caudal loop
B. Choroidal point
C. Cranial loop
D. Spinal point
E. Extradural segment

63.

What is the first branch of the external carotid artery?

A. Superior thyroid
B. Ascending pharyngeal
C. Lingual
D. Facial
E. Occipital

64.

What artery is the primary vascular supply to the nasal cavity?

A. Ophthalmic
B. Anterior ethmoidal
C. Posterior ethmoidal
D. Sphenopalatine
E. Vidian

65.

You are caring for a 42-year-old smoker who has suffered an aneurysmal subarachnoid hemorrhage. The CT findings are demonstrated below. What is the approximate risk of aneurysm rebleeding in the first 24 hours?

Use the following figure to answer questions 65 and 69:

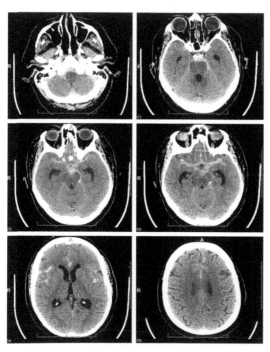

A. 4%
B. 8%
C. 12%
D. 20%
E. 33%

66.

What is the approximate risk of aneurysmal rebleed in the first 2 weeks after aneurysmal subarachnoid hemorrhage?

A. 10 to 15%
B. 15 to 20%
C. 20 to 25%
D. 25 to 30%
E. 30 to 35%

67.

Neurogenic pulmonary edema after aneurysmal subarachnoid hemorrhage is thought to occur due to what mechanism?

A. Iatrogenic fluid overload
B. Catecholamine surge
C. Heart failure
D. Pulmonary embolism
E. Prolonged mechanical ventilation

68.

What is the most common electrolyte derangement after aneurysmal subarachnoid hemorrhage?

A. Hyponatremia
B. Hypernatremia
C. Hypocalcemia
D. Hyperkalemia
E. Hypokalemia

69.

You are caring for a patient with the subarachnoid hemorrhage demonstrated in the CT scans in the Question 65. If the patient had hypernatremia, where would you suspect the underlying aneurysm to be arising from?

A. Posterior communicating artery
B. MCA bifurcation
C. Anterior communicating artery
D. Basilar tip
E. Posterior inferior cerebellar artery

70.

Which of the following helps decrease stress ulcer formation in ventilated patients with subarachnoid hemorrhage?

A. Aggressive glucose control
B. Decreasing IV infusions
C. TPN administration
D. Early enteral nutrition
E. Regular sedation holidays

71.
You are evaluating a 24-year-old woman who was an unrestrained passenger in a motor vehicle collision and she struck her head on the windshield. She was transferred to the neuro-ICU and has been intubated since admission for a depressed GCS. A pressure monitor was placed and she has evidence of refractory ICP elevations. According to the Decompressive Craniectomy in Diffuse Traumatic Brain Injury (DECRA) trial, what is the most likely outcome of decompressive hemicraniectomy in this patient?

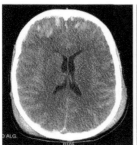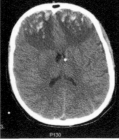

A. Mortality
B. Continued refractory ICP elevation
C. Good outcome and decreased ICP
D. Poor outcome and decreased ICP
E. Good outcome but increased ICP

72.
You are admitting an 80-year-old man to the neuro-ICU after he suffered a right-sided basal ganglia ICH with no intraventricular extension. His admission SBP is 206. According to the intensive blood pressure reduction in acute cerebral hemorrhage trial (INTERACT), intensive blood pressure control (SBP goal of 140 or less) will have what effect on this patient?

A. No change
B. Decreased hematoma volume; no clinical effect
C. Decreased hematoma volume; improved clinical course
D. Increased hematoma volume; no clinical effect
E. Increased hematoma volume; improved clinical course

73.
You are caring for a patient who has significant hypertension at baseline. Her averaged systolic blood pressure is 178 in the office. You are concerned that her blood pressure remains greater than 160, and that she has a higher risk of spontaneous ICH. What is the increased risk of ICH in patients with SBP > 160?

A. 2 times
B. 5 times
C. 10 times
D. 50 times
E. 100 times

74.
What is the rate of functional independence at 3 months in patients who suffer a spontaneous ICH?

A. 0%
B. 20%
C. 50%
D. 75%
E. 100%

75.
You are asked to consult on an 82-year-old woman with a large cerebellar hematoma from a presumed spontaneous cerebellar hemorrhage. Her admission GCS was 6 and there is evidence of intraventricular hemorrhage. The hematoma volume is measured to be 31 mL and there is brainstem compression. What is her 30-day mortality according to the ICH score?

A. 13%
B. 26%
C. 72%
D. 97%
E. 100%

76.
You are evaluating a 76-year-old woman who has suffered a right-sided spontaneous cerebral hemorrhage. The neurointensivist is asking if you would consider surgically resecting the hematoma. According to the original surgical treatment for intracerebral hemorrhage (STICH) trial subgroup analysis, what hematoma characteristic might demonstrate a benefit from surgical resection?

A. Right hemisphere location
B. Age younger than 80 years
C. Superficial cortical (< 1 cm from the surface) location
D. No midline shift
E. Intraventricular extension

77.
You are asked to evaluate the CT image of an 83-year-old woman with the following findings. What is the most common underlying cause of the findings on the CT scan?

Use the following figure to answer questions 77–79:

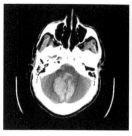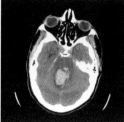

A. Hypertension
B. Age older than 80 years
C. Metastatic disease
D. Smoking
E. Drug use

78.
You are asked to discuss possible surgical outcomes with the family of a patient with the CT scan demonstrated in Question 77. When you discuss the possibility of surgical resection and decompression of the posterior fossa, they ask what chance there is that their family member can live without daily assistance. According to current literature, what is the rate of good outcome (Glasgow Outcome Score 4 or 5) in patients treated surgically for this condition?

A. 0%
B. 25%
C. 50%
D. 75%
E. 100%

79.
According to guidelines, which of the following factors present on admission should make you surgically decompress and resect the hematoma demonstrated in the CT scan in Question 77?

A. Hypertension (SBP > 160)
B. Hematoma enlargement on serial CT scan
C. GCS 15
D. Hydrocephalus
E. Elevated INR

80.
What size threshold has been identified for spontaneous cerebellar hemorrhage under which most patients are less likely to deteriorate and require surgical decompression?

A. 1 cm
B. 2 cm
C. 3 cm
D. 4 cm
E. 5 cm

81.
You performed a stereotactic needle biopsy on a 56-year-old woman who initially presented with headache and MRI demonstrated multifocal enhancement throughout the cortex. Her condition had started to worsen, and she developed cognitive impairment. The results of the biopsy are demonstrated below. What is the most likely diagnosis?

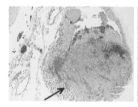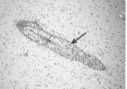

A. Glioblastoma
B. Hypertension
C. Vasculitis
D. Metastatic disease
E. Ischemic stroke

82.
What is thought to be the underlying mechanism of normal pressure hydrocephalus?

A. CSF overproduction
B. Arachnoid granulation dysfunction
C. Aqueductal stenosis
D. Multiple subclinical hemorrhages
E. Decreased ventricular compliance

83.
What diagnostic test can increase the rate of favorable response to ventriculoperitoneal (VP) shunting in patients with normal pressure hydrocephalus from approximately 50 to 80% or more?

A. Ventriculomegaly on MRI
B. Adequate CSF flow on cine MRI
C. Leukocytosis
D. Improved gait after high-volume LP
E. Perceived cognitive improvement after high-volume LP

84.
What is the diagnosis in this 18-year-old girl who presents with intermittent, right-sided holohemispheric headaches and the following MRI?

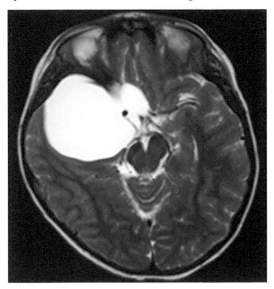

A. Pilocytic astrocytoma
B. Optic glioma
C. Epidermoid cyst
D. Arachnoid cyst
E. Metastatic disease

85.
You are caring for a 3-year-old boy who has been admitted to the pediatric ICU after nonaccidental trauma by the father that has caused severe TBI. He has elevated ICP and a poor clinical exam. The pediatric team asks you about the administration of steroids in an attempt to improve his cerebral edema. What effect do steroids have on severe pediatric TBI?

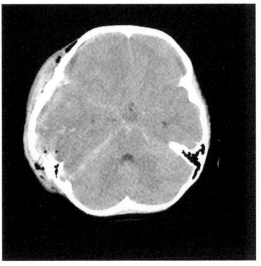

A. Improvement in ICP and clinical outcome, no systemic complications
B. Improvement in ICP and clinical outcome, increased systemic complications
C. No improvement in ICP, improved clinical outcome, increased systemic complications
D. Improvement in ICP, no clinical improvement, increased systemic complications
E. No improvement in ICP, no clinical improvement, increased systemic complications

86.
Intrauterine fetal surgery for the repair of myelomeningocele is undertaken at what time?

A. 18 to 20 weeks of gestation
B. 24 to 26 weeks of gestation
C. 30 to 32 weeks of gestation
D. 36 to 38 weeks of gestation
E. 40+ weeks of gestation

87.

You are asked to evaluate a 22-year-old woman in the ED who developed a sudden headache with some mild word-finding difficulties and admission CT is demonstrated below. She does not have any history of drug use or other systemic disease process that the ED team is currently aware of. Her INR is 1.0. What is the next best step in management?

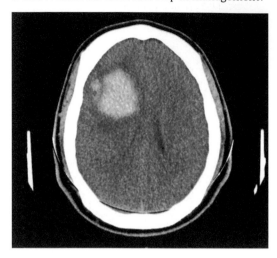

A. ICU admission and observation
B. Intensive blood pressure management
C. Intensive glucose management
D. Further imaging
E. PMR assessment

88.

You are caring for a 33-year-old man with the following lesion on cerebral angiogram. What genetic condition might predispose him to development of this lesion?

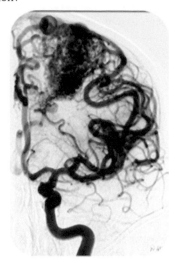

A. Neurofibromatosis type I
B. Kennedy's disease
C. Hereditary hemorrhagic telangiectasia
D. Ataxia-telangiectasia
E. Von Hippel–Lindau disease

89.

You are caring for a 38-year-old man who has been diagnosed with bilateral moyamoya disease. He has been counseled that his rate of stroke over 5 years is between 67 and 90% without treatment. He was referred to you for potential indirect or direct bypass. If your surgery is successful, what will his new rate of stroke over the next 5 years be?

A. < 10%
B. 11 to 20%
C. 21 to 30%
D. 31 to 40%
E. 41 to 50%

90.

You are evaluating a 5-year-old boy with known neurofibromatosis type I who has developed visual loss in the right eye. Imaging demonstrates a suspected right optic pathway glioma. What characteristic will determine if you are able to surgically cure this patient?

A. Baseline visual field tests
B. Optic chiasm involvement
C. Enhancement pattern on MRI
D. Location (right vs. left)
E. Patency of retinal artery on angiogram

91.
What is created when a force vector is applied tangentially and from a distance to the instantaneous axis of rotation in the spinal column?

A. Moment arm
B. Bony fracture
C. Ligamentous damage
D. Load
E. Stress shield

92.
How is the material property stress defined in spine biomechanics?

A. Change in unit length/original length
B. Force applied per unit area
C. Length of moment arm
D. Overall weight (in kg) applied to the instantaneous axis of rotation
E. Resistance of the object to deformation

93.
Stiffness of a spinal implant is defined as what?

A. The area under the force deformation curve
B. The slope of the most linear region of the force deformation curve
C. The point of maximum force on the force deformation curve
D. The point of maximum deformation on the force deformation curve

94.
On a force deformation curve, what is the term for the point where the line deflects and enters the elastic zone?

A. Fracture
B. Ultimate strength
C. Yield point
D. Preloading
E. Breaking point

95.
What percentage of patients aged 65 years will have evidence of spondylosis of the spine on imaging?

A. 10%
B. 25%
C. 50%
D. 75%
E. 95%

96.
What is thought to be the mechanism of discogenic axial back pain?

A. Facet hypertrophy and nerve root impingement
B. Disc herniation
C. Excitation of recurrent sinuvertebral nerve endings
D. Loss of disk height
E. Increased disk vascularity

97.
Small nerve fibers that innervate the facet joint have been implicated in facetogenic back pain. Where are these fibers thought to arise from?

A. Recurrent sinuvertebral nerve
B. Anterior spinal nerve ramus
C. Posterior spinal nerve ramus
D. Gray ramus communicans
E. White ramus communicans

98.
According to the National Osteoporosis Foundation guidelines, how much calcium and vitamin D should a 60-year-old woman be taking daily?

A. 400-mg calcium, 400-IU vitamin D
B. 800-mg calcium, 800-IU vitamin D
C. 1,200-mg calcium, 1,000-IU vitamin D
D. 2,000-mg calcium, 2,000-IU vitamin D
E. 3,000-mg calcium, 4,000-IU vitamin D

99.
What effect does calcitonin have?

Answer choices:

A. Inhibits osteoblasts
B. Inhibits osteoclasts
C. Promotes osteoclasts
D. Promotes osteoblasts
E. Provides structural framework for bone formation

100.
The medication raloxifene is used to prevent osteoporosis in postmenopausal women who cannot tolerate bisphosphonate therapy. It acts by inhibit osteoclasts. What side effect should patients on raloxifene be aware of?

A. Increased risk of heart attack
B. Increased risk of breast cancer
C. Increased risk of DVT
D. Increased risk of esophagitis
E. Increased bleeding tendencies

II   Answers

8 Neurosurgery

1.

B Subdural hematoma

This CT scan demonstrates an acute subdural hematoma, as evident by the hyperdense blood collection crossing the suture lines. A significant midline shift is associated. Blood remains hyperdense on CT scan for 1 to 3 days.

Further Reading: Greenberg. Handbook of Neurosurgery, 8th edition, 2016, page 895.

2.

A 1 to 3 days

This CT scan demonstrates an acute subdural hematoma, as evident by the hyperdense blood collection crossing the suture lines. A significant midline shift is associated. Blood remains hyperdense on CT scan for 1 to 3 days.

Further Reading: Greenberg. Handbook of Neurosurgery, 8th edition, 2016, page 895.

3.

D Check INR

This CT scan demonstrates an acute subdural hematoma, as evident by the hyperdense blood collection crossing the suture lines. This patient has a history of a mechanical aortic valve and is likely on chronic anticoagulation. Before you choose to intervene you should know the coagulation status of the patient and reverse if necessary.

Further Reading: Greenberg. Handbook of Neurosurgery, 8th edition, 2016, page 895.

4.

C Decompressive hemicraniotomy/ectomy

This CT scan demonstrates an acute subdural hematoma, as evident by the hyperdense blood collection crossing the suture lines. This patient will require surgery and due to the acute nature of this clot, the patient will likely not be adequately drained with burr holes. A decompressive hemicraniotomy/ectomy is recommended.

Further Reading: Greenberg. Handbook of Neurosurgery, 8th edition, 2016, page 895.

5.

C Decompressive hemicraniotomy/ectomy

This CT scan demonstrates an acute subdural hematoma, as evident by the hyperdense blood collection crossing the suture lines. According to practice guidelines in the management of acute subdural hematoma, any time the acute hematoma is > 10 mm in maximum diameter or there is > 5 mm of associated midline shift, evacuation should be performed regardless of presenting GCS.

Further Reading: Greenberg. Handbook of Neurosurgery, 8th edition, 2016, page 896.

6.

C Epidural hematoma

This CT scan demonstrates evidence of an acute epidural hematoma, as evident by the hyperdense fluid collection that does not cross the suture lines.

Further Reading: Greenberg. Handbook of Neurosurgery, 8th edition, 2016, page 892.

7.

C Foramen spinosum

This CT scan demonstrates evidence of an acute epidural hematoma, as evident by the hyperdense fluid collection that does not cross the suture lines. It is often caused by damage to the middle meningeal artery, which enters the skull through the foramen spinosum.

Further Reading: Greenberg. Handbook of Neurosurgery, 8th edition, 2016, page 892.

8.

C Operative evacuation

This CT scan demonstrates evidence of an acute epidural hematoma, as evident by the hyperdense fluid collection that does not cross the suture lines. This is a large EDH and should be evacuated emergently if possible via open surgery.

Further Reading: Greenberg. Handbook of Neurosurgery, 8th edition, 2016, page 892.

9.

B Observation/rescan

This CT scan demonstrates evidence of an acute epidural hematoma, as evident by the hyperdense fluid collection that does not cross the suture lines. This is a small epidural hematoma (< 15 mm) with less than 30 cm³ of total volume in an awake patient with an exam to follow. This patient can be observed with an early rescan to demonstrate stability in the size of the epidural hematoma. If there is significant expansion or worsening of the exam, the patient should undergo operative evacuation.

Further Reading: Greenberg. Handbook of Neurosurgery, 8th edition, 2016, page 893.

10.

D Intubate

This CT scan demonstrates evidence of an acute epidural hematoma, as evident by the hyperdense fluid collection that does not cross the suture lines. This patient had a lucid interval and has now deteriorated. Ultimately he will need operative evacuation emergently, but securing his airway should be the first priority.

Further Reading: Greenberg. Handbook of Neurosurgery, 8th edition, 2016, page 893.

11.

B Rescan in 6 hours

This patient has bifrontal contusions likely from deceleration injury to the brain parenchyma. At this point she has an exam that can be followed, but a rescan should happen after at least several hours to look for expansion of the intraparenchymal hemorrhages. They can expand in a delayed fashion and become symptomatic. A rescan should occur earlier if she deteriorates clinically.

Further Reading: Greenberg. Handbook of Neurosurgery, 8th edition, 2016, page 891.

12.

D > 3 weeks

This MRI scan demonstrates a chronic subdural hematoma. It is uniform and has a fluid appearance. This likely has been present for > 3 weeks.

Further Reading: Greenberg. Handbook of Neurosurgery, 8th edition, 2016, page 895.

13.

B Burr hole evacuation

This CT scan demonstrates a chronic subdural hematoma. It is uniform and dark in appearance. This likely has been present for > 3 weeks, and very likely can be completely drained via burr hole evacuation. It will likely not require a full craniotomy.

Further Reading: Greenberg. Handbook of Neurosurgery, 8th edition, 2016, page 895.

14.

B 15%

Approximately 15% of patients who undergo subdural fluid evacuation have a residual fluid collection at 40 days. Often times these residual collections do not require repeat surgery and can be managed with observation and serial CT examinations.

Further Reading: Greenberg. Handbook of Neurosurgery, 8th edition, 2016, page 901.

15.

C Biventricular trajectory

Dating back to initial research done by Harvey Cushing and further studied recently, it has been demonstrated that biventricular trajectory through the third ventricle is uniformly fatal in the civilian literature. Bifrontal, holohemispheric, and isolated cerebellar trajectories have not been found to be uniformly fatal.

Further Reading: Greenberg. Handbook of Neurosurgery, 8th edition, 2016, page 911.

16.

C Tension pneumocephalus

This CT scan demonstrates tension pneumocephalus, the classic "Mount Fuji" sign. This is not a fluid collection given how dark the findings are on CT scan and can only be air.

Further Reading: Greenberg. Handbook of Neurosurgery, 8th edition, 2016, page 888.

17.

A Decompression

This CT scan demonstrates tension pneumocephalus, the classic "Mount Fuji" sign. This patient is symptomatic from this air collection and while the CSF leak certainly needs to be repaired, the patient should have some form of decompression of the pressurized gas within the skull, followed shortly thereafter by repair of the CSF leak.

Further Reading: Greenberg. Handbook of Neurosurgery, 8th edition, 2016, page 889.

18.

B No

This player has evidence of a concussion, including disorientation and amnesia to the event. Based on current concussion guidelines, this player should be removed from the game and not allowed to return until evaluated further by a licensed healthcare provider trained in evaluating concussions.

Further Reading: Greenberg. Handbook of Neurosurgery, 8th edition, 2016, page 844.

19.

C 10 to 15

Normal ICP range for adults and older children is 10 to 15 mm Hg. Young children generally range from 3 to 7 mm Hg, and infants range from 1.5 to 6 mm Hg.

Further Reading: Greenberg. Handbook of Neurosurgery, 8th edition, 2016, page 857.

20.

C CPP = MAP − ICP

Cerebral perfusion pressure is calculated by subtracting the intracranial pressure from the mean arterial pressure. Based on autoregulation, the brain can maintain normal cerebral blood flow at a wide range of CPP, generally between 50 and 150 mm Hg.

Further Reading: Greenberg. Handbook of Neurosurgery, 8th edition, 2016, page 857.

21.

C Operative elevation/debridement

This patient has evidence of a depressed skull fracture with an underlying hematoma. Given the concerning underlying hematoma and depth of the depressed skull fracture segment, this fracture should be elevated and the hematoma should be addressed surgically.

Further Reading: Greenberg. Handbook of Neurosurgery, 8th edition, 2016, page 882.

22.

A Longitudinal

There are two types of temporal bone fractures, longitudinal and transverse. Longitudinal fractures are parallel to the EAC and are the most common type of temporal bone fractures. The longitudinal fracture does not tend to put stretch forces on the geniculate ganglion and therefore is less likely to lead to VII nerve injury.

Further Reading: Greenberg. Handbook of Neurosurgery, 8th edition, 2016, page 884.

23.

B Transverse

There are two types of temporal bone fractures, longitudinal and transverse. Transverse fractures are perpendicular to the EAC and are the less common type of temporal bone fractures (20–30%). The transverse fracture tends to pass through the cochlea and can put stretch forces on the geniculate ganglion leading to VII nerve injury.

Further Reading: Greenberg. Handbook of Neurosurgery, 8th edition, 2016, page 884.

24.

C Start steroids

With a transverse temporal bone fracture, VII nerve injury can occur. While efficacy is currently unproven, many surgeons will start glucocorticoids in the presence of facial nerve dysfunction in the setting of a transverse temporal bone fracture. ENT consultation should be considered as decompression may be required if facial nerve function does not improve.

Further Reading: Greenberg. Handbook of Neurosurgery, 8th edition, 2016, page 884.

25.

B NG tube insertion

Clival fractures are severe injuries that are often fatal. They can be associated with cranial nerve deficits, diabetes insipidus, and anterior/posterior circulation vascular injury. NG tube insertion should be avoided as there have been reports of intracranial NG tube insertion through a diastased fracture of the clivus.

Further Reading: Greenberg. Handbook of Neurosurgery, 8th edition, 2016, page 885.

26.

C Type III

There are three types of Lefort facial fractures, and of these, type III involves the zygomatic arches, the nasofrontal suture, and orbital floors. Given the type of fracture and the forces required, there is a high incidence of brain injury with type III Lefort fractures.

Further Reading: Greenberg. Handbook of Neurosurgery, 8th edition, 2016, page 887.

27.

B Observation

In a neurologically normal infant, this fracture should be managed nonoperatively. This is the classic "ping-pong" fracture, and over time the CSF pulsations will remodel the bone and heal this fracture. Operative intervention is generally not required.

Further Reading: Greenberg. Handbook of Neurosurgery, 8th edition, 2016, page 915.

28.

A Growing skull fracture

This CT scan demonstrates widening of the skull fracture with evidence of fluid below the fracture. This is consistent with a growing skull fracture, and is often seen with a dural laceration and CSF leak that goes unrepaired. It is different than an arachnoid cyst and should be managed operatively with dural closure.

Further Reading: Greenberg. Handbook of Neurosurgery, 8th edition, 2016, page 915.

29.

D Circumferential craniotomy and dural repair

This CT scan demonstrates widening of the skull fracture with evidence of fluid below the fracture. This is consistent with a growing skull fracture, and is often seen with a dural laceration and CSF leak that goes unrepaired. It is different than an arachnoid cyst and should be managed operatively with dural closure.

Further Reading: Greenberg. Handbook of Neurosurgery, 8th edition, 2016, page 915.

30.

B Bilateral subdural hematomas

Suspected non-accidental trauma workup should include some form of intracranial injury. When a child is shaken, bilateral subdural hematomas can develop due to shear forces exerted on the brain leading to tearing of bridging veins.

Further Reading: Greenberg. Handbook of Neurosurgery, 8th edition, 2016, page 916.

31.

A Nonaccidental trauma

While all options listed can cause retinal hemorrhages, nonaccidental trauma is the most common cause seen in an infant. 16/26 battered children < 3 years of age had RH on fundoscopy, while 1/32 nonbattered children with head injury had RH. The single false positive was due to traumatic parturition.

Further Reading: Greenberg. Handbook of Neurosurgery, 8th edition, 2016, page 916.

32.

B GFAP

GFAP, a marker of neurons, has been shown to be associated with acute traumatic brain injury and may be used in the future to determine which patients need to undergo CT scan of the brain.

Further Reading: Brain injury biomarkers may improve the predictive power of the IMPACT outcome calculator. J Neurotrauma. 2012, 1770–1778.

33.

A Continued medical management

According to the initial results of the DECRA trial, decompressive hemicraniectomy in the setting of elevated ICP in patients < 60 years of age within 72 hours of injury refractory to first line medical management was associated with a higher rate of unfavorable outcome than the control group who did not undergo surgery. In a subgroup analysis, there was no difference when patients who had bilaterally unreactive pupils were controlled for (initial analysis had significantly higher rate of bilaterally unreactive pupils in the surgical arm). While some providers would perform a decompression, strictly according to the results of the DECRA trial, this will lead to unfavorable outcomes. Further surgical trials are underway, and results depend on the definition of favorable outcome.

Further Reading: Kolias AG. Traumatic brain injury in adults. Pract Neurol. 2013, 228–235.

34.

C Drilling to the floor of the middle fossa

It is important to ensure that a decompressive craniectomy is large enough to not only decompress the cerebral hemisphere, but to also avoid complications that have been shown to occur when the AP diameter of the craniectomy is < 12 cm. Subsequent herniation of the brain can, through the craniectomy defect, lead to vascular injury and further infarction of the brain. When uncal herniation is suspected, making sure the craniectomy reaches the floor of the middle fossa is important to fully decompress the temporal lobe.

Further Reading: Wagner S. Suboptimum hemicraniectomy as a cause of additional cerebral lesions in patients with malignant infarction of the MCA. J Neurosurg. 2001, 693–696.

35.

A Hypotension

Cushing's triad is seen often during terminal elevation of ICP immediately before herniation. It consists of bradycardia, hypertension, and breathing irregularities. If these findings are seen together in a patient with elevated ICP, action should be taken immediately to decrease ICP as the patient is likely about to herniate.

Further Reading: Greenberg. Handbook of Neurosurgery, 8th edition, 2016, page 858.

36.

B ~ 30 minutes

CO_2 is a potent vasodilator and hyperventilation can be used to decrease intracranial pressure by decreasing CO_2. The brain is able to buffer efficiently, and therefore this technique may only transiently decrease ICP as the brain will adjust to new levels of CO_2 within 20 to 30 minutes.

Further Reading: Greenberg. Handbook of Neurosurgery, 8th edition, 2016, page 868.

37.

D 31 to 35 mm Hg

CO_2 is a potent vasodilator and hyperventilation can be used to decrease intracranial pressure by decreasing CO_2. The brain is able to buffer efficiently, and therefore this technique may only transiently decrease ICP as the brain will adjust to new levels of CO_2 within 20 to 30 minutes. You are aiming for a $PaCO_2$ of 31 to 35 mm Hg.

Further Reading: Greenberg. Handbook of Neurosurgery, 8th edition, 2016, page 868.

38.

D 324

Mannitol is a very effective osmotic diuretic that is often used to decrease intracranial pressure. When utilized in a scheduled fashion, monitoring of serum osmolality should take place. When serum osmolality is greater than 320, other options should be considered for medical treatment of raised ICP.

Further Reading: Greenberg. Handbook of Neurosurgery, 8th edition, 2016, page 868.

39.

B 11 cm back from the nasion, mid-pupillary line

Kocher's point is thought to be located generally between 10.5 and 11.5 cm back from the nasion and roughly 3 to 3.5 cm lateral, or in the mid-pupillary line. Generally speaking this is a good location to place a burr hole for an EVD placement for acute hydrocephalus. In many situations, simply placing the EVD perpendicular to the skull will lead to ventricular puncture, depending on ventricular size.

Further Reading: Citow, Macdonald, Refai. Comprehensive Neurosurgery Board Review, 2nd edition, 2010, page 473.

40.

B 3%

Hypertonic saline can be used for ICP management either as a first line agent or in patient's refractory to mannitol administration. The patient can be given 3% saline as a continuous infusion through a peripheral IV, but 7% and 23.4% given as a bolus should be administered through a central line to avoid deleterious effects to the extremities.

Further Reading: Greenberg. Handbook of Neurosurgery, 8th edition, 2016, page 875.

41.

B 150 mL

The approximate volume of CSF in the system is 150 mL at any given time. Roughly 450 to 500 mL of CSF is produced each day, and the CSF turns over 3 times daily.

Further Reading: Greenberg. Handbook of Neurosurgery, 8th edition, 2016, page 856.

42.

B 10

This patient has a GCS of 10. E = 2, V = 3, M = 5.

Further Reading: Citow, Macdonald, Refai. Comprehensive Neurosurgery Board Review, 2nd edition, 2010, page 496.

43.

A 4t

This patient has a GCS of 4t. E = 1, V = 1t, M = 2. This patient is decerebrate posturing (M = 2), is not opening his eyes (E = 1), and is intubated (V = 1t).

Further Reading: Citow, Macdonald, Refai. Comprehensive Neurosurgery Board Review, 2nd edition, 2010, page 496.

44.

C 13.6 cm H_2O

There is a lack of convention among neurosurgeons as to what system should be utilized, mm Hg or cm H_2O. 1 mm Hg = 1.36 cm H_2O, meaning that 10 mm Hg = 13.6 cm H_2O.

Further Reading: Greenberg. Handbook of Neurosurgery. 8th edition, 2016, page 861.

45.

A Lundberg A waves

There are three types of Lundberg waves seen during ICP monitoring: A, B, and C. Lundberg A (plateau waves) are associated with extremely high elevation of ICP that plateaus for 5 to 20 minutes and then decreases to ~ 20 mm Hg for 30 to 45 minutes followed by another elevation. MAP increases can be seen as well. These waves are not often seen in the ICU setting as active ICP management is taking place.

Further Reading: Greenberg. Handbook of Neurosurgery. 8th edition, 2016, page 865.

46.

B P2

The second ICP wave, P2, represents the pressure when the aortic pulse bounces off the ventricular wall (P1 is the aortic pulse itself). When the ventricular walls are stiffened due to hydrocephalus and lack compliance, the P2 wave will be greatly increased and will lead to the classic ICP waveform that is indicative of elevated ICP.

Further Reading: Greenberg. Handbook of Neurosurgery. 8th edition, 2016, page 864.

47.

B > 50

Cerebral perfusion pressure is calculated by subtracting ICP from the mean arterial pressure. The brain can autoregulate CPP to maintain stable cerebral blood flow at 55 to 60 mL/100 mg/min. This autoregulation curve in a normal brain keeps flow stable between CPPs of 50 and 150.

Further Reading: Greenberg. Handbook of Neurosurgery. 8th edition, 2016, page 869.

48.

B 85

Cerebral perfusion pressure is calculated by subtracting ICP from the mean arterial pressure. The brain can autoregulate CPP to maintain stable cerebral blood flow at 55 to 60 mL/100 mg/min. This autoregulation curve in a normal brain keeps flow stable between CPPs of 50 and 150. It is thought during severe TBI that autoregulation fails and that CBF matches CPP much more closely. In this setting, an MAP of 85 with an ICP of 25 will give you a CPP of 60, exactly matching the standard CBF of the brain in normal conditions.

Further Reading: Greenberg. Handbook of Neurosurgery. 8th edition, 2016, page 869.

49.

B 3

This patient has a GCS of 3t. E = 1, V = 1t, M = 1. GCS of 0 is not possible. You get 3 points just for showing up.

Further Reading: Citow, Macdonald, Refai. Comprehensive Neurosurgery Board Review, 2nd edition, 2010, page 496.

50.

D Pentobarbital

Pentobarbital is a last resort medical management strategy for reducing raised ICP. It provides maximal reduction in $CMRO_2$ and CBF when compared to other agents, but should be used as a last resort. It should be titrated to burst suppression on EEG. It can cause severe hypotension and paralytic ileus. It also stores within fat deposits so dosing should be adjusted. It can confound any attempts at brain death examination until it has been completely metabolized from the system, which can take days.

Further Reading: Greenberg. Handbook of Neurosurgery, 8th edition, 2016, page 875.

51.

C Awake language mapping

This imaging demonstrates a left frontal likely low grade astrocytoma of the frontal region. This should concern you for potential involvement of Broca's area, and may make you consider performing the procedure awake with language mapping.

Further Reading: Bernstein, Berger. Neuro-Oncology: The Essentials. 3rd edition, 2015, page 160.

52.

C Functional MRI

This MRI demonstrates a left frontal likely low grade astrocytoma frontal region. This should concern you for potential involvement of Broca's area, and you could consider performing an fMRI to localize language structures prior to surgical decision making.

Further Reading: Bernstein, Berger. Neuro-Oncology: The Essentials. 3rd edition, 2015, page 160.

53.

A Motor mapping

This MRI demonstrates a likely anaplastic astrocytoma of the posterior frontal lobe on the right. There is concern that this tumor involves the motor strip and thus intraoperative motor mapping could be useful during this resection.

Further Reading: Bernstein, Berger. Neuro-Oncology: The Essentials. 3rd edition, 2015, page 160.

54.

C Phase reversal

When motor mapping for tumor resection near the motor strip, you are looking for phase reversal of the signal on monitoring. This shows the change from the sensory cortex to the motor cortex.

Further Reading: Bernstein, Berger. Neuro-Oncology: The Essentials. 3rd edition, 2015, page 160.

55.

D 5

These intraoperative recordings demonstrate phase reversal between electrodes 3 and 5. This means that in this scenario the motor strip is likely located under electrode 5. Electrode 4 is very likely located directly over the central sulcus, given the lack of response.

Further Reading: Bernstein, Berger. Neuro-Oncology: The Essentials. 3rd edition, 2015, page 160.

56.

B Metastases

Metastases are the most common tumor of the central nervous system, and account for just over 50% of intracranial tumors.

Further Reading: Bernstein, Berger. Neuro-Oncology: The Essentials. 3rd edition, 2015, page 451.

57.

B Lung

Overall, lung cancer has the highest incidence of brain metastases based on autopsy data currently available.

Further Reading: Greenberg. Handbook of Neurosurgery. 8th edition, 2016, page 801.

Bernstein, Berger. Neuro-Oncology: The Essentials. 3rd edition, 2015, page 451.

58.

D Breast

Breast cancer metastases are the most common metastatic tumor to the brain in females.

Further Reading: Schouten LJ. Incidence of brain metastases in a cohort of patients with carcinoma of the breast, colon, kidney, lung and melanoma. Cancer. 2002.

Bernstein, Berger. Neuro-Oncology: The Essentials. 3rd edition, 2015, page 451.

59.

B CT chest, abdomen, and pelvis

This MRI demonstrates evidence of metastatic disease. In a patient with no prior history of primary cancer, workup should proceed with a CT CAP to look for primary disease.

Further Reading: Bernstein, Berger. Neuro-Oncology: The Essentials. 3rd edition, 2015, page 451.

60.

B Renal cell carcinoma

Renal cell carcinoma has a higher propensity for hemorrhagic conversion of a cerebral metastatic lesion.

Further Reading: Greenberg. Handbook of Neurosurgery. 8th edition, 2016, page 805.

Bernstein, Berger. Neuro-Oncology: The Essentials. 3rd edition, 2015, page 451.

61.

A Multiple myeloma

Of the tumor types listed here, multiple myeloma is radiosensitive. The other lesions are highly resistant.

Further Reading: Greenberg. Handbook of Neurosurgery. 8th edition, 2016, page 809.

62.

D Renal cell carcinoma

Of the tumor types listed here, renal cell carcinoma is highly resistant to radiation. The other lesions are considered radiosensitive to varying degrees.

Further Reading: Greenberg. Handbook of Neurosurgery. 8th edition, 2016, page 809.

63.

A 70

KPS is used to determine patient function in follow-up for many tumor resections. A KPS of 70 or greater means the patient is able to at least care for himself or herself without assistance.

Further Reading: Greenberg. Handbook of Neurosurgery. 8th edition, 2016, page 1358.

64.

A Surgical resection

In patients with a single brain met (of any type) with a KPS > 70 and no evidence of extra cranial disease, surgery plus radiation increased median survival by 25 weeks. Surgical resection should be offered in this case in order to obtain tissue diagnosis if no primary can be found.

Further Reading: Greenberg. Handbook of Neurosurgery. 8th edition, 2016, page 804.

65.

B Leptomeninges

Melanocytes are found in the leptomeninges and are thought to be the probable origination point for primary CNS melanoma.

Further Reading: Greenberg. Handbook of Neurosurgery. 8th edition, 2016, page 701.

66.

B 33%

Nearly 33% of patients with incidentally discovered meningiomas will exhibit no growth over a 3-year follow-up period. Many of these patients can simply be observed depending on symptomatology.

Further Reading: Greenberg. Handbook of Neurosurgery. 8th edition, 2016, page 690.

67.

B Arachnoid cap cells

Meningiomas arise from arachnoid cap cells of the CNS. They can arise from wherever these arachnoid cap cells are found, including between the brain and skull, ventricles, and surrounding the spinal cord.

Further Reading: Greenberg. Handbook of Neurosurgery. 8th edition, 2016, page 690.

68.

A ~ 1 to 3%

Meningiomas are thought to have roughly 1 to 3% incidence in the general population > 60 years of age based on autopsy studies.

Further Reading: Greenberg. Handbook of Neurosurgery. 8th edition, 2016, page 690.

69.

B Parasagittal

Parasagittal meningiomas are thought to be the most common location, followed by convexity meningiomas, based on a series of 336 cases.

Further Reading: Greenberg. Handbook of Neurosurgery. 8th edition, 2016, page 691.

70.

C Olfactory groove meningioma

Foster-Kennedy syndrome (anosmia, ipsilateral optic atrophy, and contralateral papilledema) was classically described in the setting of an olfactory groove meningioma.

Further Reading: Greenberg. Handbook of Neurosurgery. 8th edition, 2016, page 691.

71.

D Fibrillary

Fibrillary astrocytoma is the most common subtype of WHO grade II astrocytoma.

Further Reading: Greenberg. Handbook of Neurosurgery. 8th edition, 2016, page 615.

72.

D Surgical resection

Surgical resection is considered the principal treatment for low-grade gliomas to both establish the diagnosis and for cytoreduction. More aggressive surgical excision has been shown to be associated with better outcome and further time to malignant transformation. XRT and chemotherapy may follow later in the disease course.

Further Reading: Greenberg. Handbook of Neurosurgery. 8th edition, 2016, page 620.

73.

C 5-year increase in progression-free survival

In subtotally resected low-grade gliomas, 54 Gy XRT has been associated with an increased PFS from 3.4 to 5.3 years and is recommended as an early adjuvant treatment.

Further Reading: Greenberg. Handbook of Neurosurgery. 8th edition, 2016, page 620.

74.

A No difference in progression-free survival

In gross totally resected low-grade gliomas, 54 Gy XRT has been associated with no increase in PFS and should be deferred until progression occurs.

Further Reading: Greenberg. Handbook of Neuro-surgery. 8th edition, 2016, page 620.

75.

E > 97%

Extent of resection matters when undergoing attempted gross total resection of a GBM. Extent of resection > 97% has been shown to be associated with prolonged overall survival.

Further Reading: Greenberg. Handbook of Neuro-surgery. 8th edition, 2016, page 621.

76.

D 60 Gy XRT + temozolomide chemotherapy

The Stupp regimen of chemoradiation for GBM consists of 60 Gy XRT in fractions along with con-current TMZ and adjuvant chemotherapy. PCV chemotherapy was attempted, but showed no benefit in an RCT prior to publication of the Stupp regimen.

Further Reading: Greenberg. Handbook of Neuro-surgery. 8th edition, 2016, page 622.

77.

B 14.6 months

The Stupp regimen of chemoradiation for GBM consists of 60 Gy XRT in fractions along with con-current TMZ and adjuvant chemotherapy. In the classic article, median survival increased from 12.1 months to 14.6 months.

Further Reading: Greenberg. Handbook of Neuro-surgery. 8th edition, 2016, page 622.

78.

B 10.8 months

The Stupp regimen of chemoradiation for GBM consists of 60 Gy XRT in fractions along with con-current TMZ and adjuvant chemotherapy. In the classic article, median survival increased from 12.1 months to 14.6 months. When a subgroup of patients with MGMT promoter methylation was studied, it was found that these patients had a me-dian survival of 23.4 months compared to 12.6 in non–MGMT methylated patients, leading to a me-dian overall survival benefit of 10.8 months.

Further Reading: Greenberg. Handbook of Neuro-surgery. 8th edition, 2016, page 622.

79.

B Myelosuppression

The main side effect of TMZ chemotherapy is myelosuppression, and it is an otherwise well tolerated chemotherapeutic. Patients undergo routine neutrophil testing and should have a neu-trophil count of > 1.5 × 10^9/L and a platelet count > 100.

Further Reading: Greenberg. Handbook of Neuro-surgery. 8th edition, 2016, page 622.

80.

C Pseudoprogression

In MGMT promoter methylated GBM patients, contrast enhancement can be seen at roughly 3 months post gross total resection and Stupp reg-imen. It is consistent with pseudoprogression and often decreases on subsequent imaging and symp-toms can resolve with steroids. It is associated with radiation kill of the tumor. At this time there are no definitive imaging studies that can prove pseu-doprogression vs tumor recurrence, but this is an active area of research.

Further Reading: Greenberg. Handbook of Neuro-surgery. 8th edition, 2016, page 623.

81.

D Myelosuppression

Bevacizumab is a monoclonal antibody against VEGF and is FDA approved for the treatment of recurrent GBM. Its side effect profile consists of hypertension, arterial thromboembolism, hemor-rhage, GI perforations, wound healing complica-tions, and fistula formation.

Further Reading: Greenberg. Handbook of Neuro-surgery. 8th edition, 2016, page 624.

82.

A 1 to 20 years

Pilocytic astrocytoma is a WHO grade I tumor with a predilection for younger patients. Approxi-mately 75% of these tumors present in patients less than 20 years of age.

Further Reading: Greenberg. Handbook of Neuro-surgery. 8th edition, 2016, page 630.

83.

A Observation

Pilocytic astroyctomas in the pediatric popula-tion that are incompletely resected should be initial-ly observed as the rate of growth over 5, 10, or even 20 years can be minimal. Radiation and chemother-apy should be saved for obvious recurrence with growth demonstrated on serial imaging studies.

Further Reading: Greenberg. Handbook of Neuro-surgery. 8th edition, 2016, page 631.

84.

D Patients age at diagnosis + 9 months

Collins' law suggests that pediatric patients with pilocytic astrocytomas can be considered cured if there is no recurrence after enough time has passed adding the patient's age at time of diagnosis + 9 months. It is controversial, but often quoted.

Further Reading: Greenberg. Handbook of Neurosurgery. 8th edition, 2016, page 631.

85.

B Optic glioma

Optic gliomas are found in patients with neurofibromatosis and often present with unilateral painless proptosis. Visual loss occurs when the glioma has reached the chiasm or is causing significant mass effect on the optic nerve. These lesions can be cured if complete excision of the optic nerve and eye occur before the tumor has invaded the optic chiasm.

Further Reading: Greenberg. Handbook of Neurosurgery. 8th edition, 2016, page 632.

86.

D Observation

This MRI demonstrates diffuse enlargement of the brainstem consistent with a diffuse intrinsic pontine glioma. Diagnosis can often be made based on MRI scans and surgical resection/biopsy should be avoided unless an obvious exophytic component is present. Children with this diagnosis die within 6 to 12 months, and XRT may not prolong survival.

Further Reading: Greenberg. Handbook of Neurosurgery. 8th edition, 2016, page 634.

87.

B Temporal lobe

PXAs tend to occur in the temporal lobe, are cystic with an enhancing nodule, and present with seizures.

Further Reading: Greenberg. Handbook of Neurosurgery. 8th edition, 2016, page 636.

88.

C PCV chemotherapy alone

For pathology proven oligodendrogliomas, postoperative PCV chemotherapy has shown to be beneficial. XRT is controversial, and often saved for malignant transformation or recurrent growth. At this time immediate XRT post-resection is not often recommended.

Further Reading: Greenberg. Handbook of Neurosurgery. 8th edition, 2016, page 640.

89.

C Facial weakness

Ependymomas often present in the fourth ventricle, originating from the floor of the fourth ventricle. Given their invasiveness, they may involve the facial colliculus which is located in the floor of the fourth ventricle, making facial weakness a likely cranial nerve deficit. Lateral rectus palsy (CN VI involvement) can be seen as well.

Further Reading: Greenberg. Handbook of Neurosurgery. 8th edition, 2016, page 643.

90.

C MRI spinal axis

Ependymomas often present in the fourth ventricle, originating from the floor of the fourth ventricle. They can cause drop metastases within the spinal canal, and thus MRI imaging of the entire neuraxis should be performed prior to intervention.

Further Reading: Greenberg. Handbook of Neurosurgery. 8th edition, 2016, page 644.

91.

C XRT alone

Ependymomas often present in the fourth ventricle, originating from the floor of the fourth ventricle. They tend to be radiosensitive and have not been shown to benefit from added chemotherapy. Traditional XRT therapy included 45 to 48 Gy to the tumor bed with 15 to 20 Gy reserved for recurrence. With the development of 3D conformal XRT, doses of 59.4 Gy to the tumor bed have been given. Prophylactic spinal XRT is usually given only if there is evidence of drop metastases on imaging.

Further Reading: Greenberg. Handbook of Neurosurgery. 8th edition, 2016, page 644.

92.

B Central neurocytoma

Central neurocytomas are WHO grade II neuronal tumors often found attached to the septum pellucidum in the frontal horn of the lateral ventricles.

Further Reading: Greenberg. Handbook of Neurosurgery. 8th edition, 2016, page 645.

93.

C Third ventricle

Gelastic seizures are characterized by inappropriate laughter and are often seen with hypothalamic hamartomas or hypothalamic gliomas with a mass in the third ventricle.

Further Reading: Baltuch, Villemure. Operative Techniques in Epilepsy Surgery, 2009, page 83.

94.

D Observation

DNETs are often seen in the temporal lobe and appear to have nodular enhancement on MRI. They are WHO grade I tumors and are associated with medically intractable epilepsy. After gross total resection, observation is recommended as XRT and chemotherapy have not shown any benefit in these benign tumors.

Further Reading: Greenberg. Handbook of Neurosurgery. 8th edition, 2016, page 647.

95.

A Cardiac arrhythmia

Paraganglioma (glomus tumors) can secrete epinephrine and norepinephrine based on histologic subtype, and therefore aggressive manipulation can lead to release of these catecholamines and hypertension/cardiac arrhythmias may occur.

Further Reading: Greenberg. Handbook of Neurosurgery. 8th edition, 2016, page 653.

96.

D Carotid body tumor

Carotid body tumor is the most common paraganglioma of the ones listed here. Overall, pheochromocytoma is the most common paraganglioma.

Further Reading: Greenberg. Handbook of Neurosurgery. 8th edition, 2016, page 653.

97.

A Sympathetic ganglion

Neuroblastomas are aggressive tumors that arise from the sympathetic ganglion. They often present in the adrenal gland (40%), but can present anywhere along the sympathetic chain and in certain presentations can cause a Horner's syndrome.

Further Reading: Greenberg. Handbook of Neurosurgery. 8th edition, 2016, page 657.

98.

B Choriocarcinoma

CSF markers are important for pineal region tumors. In this case there is an isolated elevation of B-HCG which leads to the diagnosis of choriocarcinoma.

Further Reading: Greenberg. Handbook of Neurosurgery. 8th edition, 2016, page 660.

99.

A Germinoma

CSF markers are important for pineal region tumors. In this case there is elevation of both B-HCG and placental alkaline phosphatase (PLAP), which is suggestive of germinoma. While PLAP is often positive in germinomas, B-HCG has been shown to be positive in 10 to 50% of cases based on the microarchitecture of the tumor and whether or not syncytiotrophoblasts are present.

Further Reading: Greenberg. Handbook of Neurosurgery. 8th edition, 2016, page 660.

100.

D Mature teratoma

CSF markers are important for pineal region tumors. In this case, the markers are all negative, and this can be the case with a mixed germ cell tumor or a mature teratoma.

Further Reading: Greenberg. Handbook of Neurosurgery. 8th edition, 2016, page 660.

101.

C Embryonal carcinoma

CSF markers are important for pineal region tumors. In this case, AFP is elevated while the other markers are negative. This is suggestive of embryonal carcinoma, yolk sac carcinoma, or immature teratoma.

Further Reading: Greenberg. Handbook of Neurosurgery. 8th edition, 2016, page 660.

102.

B Facial numbness

Patients with vestibular schwannomas are actually more likely to present with facial numbness than weakness. Often times the facial nerve is distorted by the tumor but no weakness is present. However, with fairly minor compression of the trigeminal nerve, facial numbness can occur. This is likely due to resiliency of motor nerves compared to sensory nerves.

Further Reading: Greenberg. Handbook of Neurosurgery. 8th edition, 2016, page 671.

103.

D Hearing loss

Unilateral hearing loss is overall the most common presentation of vestibular schwannomas.

Further Reading: Greenberg. Handbook of Neurosurgery. 8th edition, 2016, page 672.

104.

C Observation

In patients with a vestibular schwannoma < 15 mm in size with intact hearing, observation with serial scans every 6 months should be the initial next step. If/when tumor growth is documented > 2 mm, treatment is recommended.

Further Reading: Greenberg. Handbook of Neurosurgery. 8th edition, 2016, page 676.

105.

A Anterior

The facial nerve is displaced anteriorly in up to 75% of cases, but can also be seen superiorly displaced. It can be completely thinned out over the surface of the tumor, so monitoring is recommended.

Further Reading: Greenberg. Handbook of Neurosurgery. 8th edition, 2016, page 679.

106.

A 20%

Hemangioblastomas can be associated with VHL, but can also occur sporadically. They seem to be associated with VHL approximately 20% of the time.

Further Reading: Greenberg. Handbook of Neurosurgery. 8th edition, 2016, page 701.

107.

C Paraganglioma

VHL is a disease associated with abnormalities on chromosome 3. It is associated with multiple tumor types including hemangioblastomas, retinal hemangioblastomas, pheochromocytomas, renal cell carcinoma, cystadenomas, pancreactic neuroendocrine tumors, and endolymphatic sac tumors.

Further Reading: Greenberg. Handbook of Neurosurgery. 8th edition, 2016, page 705.

108.

B XRT + methotrexate chemotherapy

Primary CNS lymphoma that is non-AIDS related and biopsy proven is best treated with XRT and methotrexate chemotherapy. There is no role for surgical debulking as this has demonstrated no improvement in survival in this patient population.

Further Reading: Greenberg. Handbook of Neurosurgery. 8th edition, 2016, page 713.

109.

A 3 to 4%

Primary CNS lymphoma that is non-AIDS related and biopsy proven is best treated with XRT and methotrexate chemotherapy. There is no role for surgical debulking as this has demonstrated no improvement in survival in this patient population. Approximate 5-year survival is 3 to 4%.

Further Reading: Greenberg. Handbook of Neurosurgery. 8th edition, 2016, page 713.

110.

B > 1 cm

Pituitary adenomas are considered macroadenomas after they have grown to >1 cm in size.

Further Reading: Greenberg. Handbook of Neurosurgery. 8th edition, 2016, page 718.

111.

D 65%

Approximately 65% of pituitary tumors secrete an active hormone, with prolactin being the most commonly secreted hormone (48%), followed by growth hormone (10%), ACTH (6%), and TSH (1%).

Further Reading: Greenberg. Handbook of Neurosurgery. 8th edition, 2016, page 719.

112.

D Bitemporal hemianopia

Pituitary macroadenomas cause compression of the optic chiasm and given their midline location lead to bitemporal hemianopia.

Further Reading: Greenberg. Handbook of Neurosurgery. 8th edition, 2016, page 720.

113.

C Sodium

Suprasellar germinomas can lead to compression of the pituitary stalk and lead to diabetes insipidus. With elevated serum sodium in a suprasellar mass, germinoma should be considered.

Further Reading: Schwartz, Anand. Endoscopic Pituitary Surgery, 2012, page 53.

114.

B Visual field cut

Pituitary apoplexy occurs when a pituitary tumor hemorrhages into the sella. These patients often need emergent corticosteroid administration, but progressive visual field deficit is a reason to emergently decompress the sella. This should ideally be performed within 7 days of onset to promote full recovery.

Further Reading: Greenberg. Handbook of Neurosurgery. 8th edition, 2016, page 721.

115.

A Cushing's disease

Cushing's syndrome describes the general features of hypercortisolism, whereas Cushing's disease is Cushing's syndrome caused by an ACTH secreting pituitary adenoma.

Further Reading: Greenberg. Handbook of Neurosurgery. 8th edition, 2016, page 723.

116.

C Nelson's syndrome

Nelson's syndrome occurs when ACTH producing pituitary adenoma cells remain after bilateral adrenalectomy for Cushing's disease. Given the cross-reactivity between ACTH and melanocyte stimulating hormone, patients notice hyperpigmentation and signs/symptoms of an enlarging pituitary mass. She should undergo surgical resection of the mass.

Further Reading: Greenberg. Handbook of Neurosurgery. 8th edition, 2016, page 725.

117.

B Colon cancer

Patients with growth hormone–secreting tumors and acromegaly have a two times increased risk of colon cancer compared to the normal population.

Further Reading: Greenberg. Handbook of Neurosurgery. 8th edition, 2016, page 726.

118.

B D2 dopamine receptor

The main medication used for prolactinomas currently is cabergoline, a D2 receptor agonist, compared to bromocriptine which is a nonselective (D1 and D2) dopamine agonist.

Further Reading: Greenberg. Handbook of Neurosurgery. 8th edition, 2016, page 740.

119.

C Mitral regurgitation

The main medication used for prolactinomas currently is cabergoline, a D2 receptor agonist, and it can lead to cardiac valve regurgitation.

Further Reading: Greenberg. Handbook of Neurosurgery. 8th edition, 2016, page 740.

120.

C Somatostatin analogue

While many growth hormone–secreting pituitary adenomas can be treated with surgery, occasionally medical management is attempted using octreotide, which is a somatostatin analogue. Tumor volume decreases in approximately 30% of patients.

Further Reading: Greenberg. Handbook of Neurosurgery. 8th edition, 2016, page 742.

121.

A GH receptor antagonist

While many growth hormone–secreting pituitary adenomas can be treated with surgery, occasionally medical management is attempted using pegvisomant, which is a growth hormone receptor antagonist. In patients treated for 12 months, normal IGF levels are seen in 97% of patients, but tumor size remains the same.

Further Reading: Greenberg. Handbook of Neurosurgery. 8th edition, 2016, page 742.

122.

B Garnder's syndrome

Gardner's syndrome is comprised of colonic polyposis, multiple cranial osteomas, and soft tissue tumors. Osteomas of the skull consist of osteoid tissue within osteoblastic tissue with reactive bone formation around that region.

Further Reading: Greenberg. Handbook of Neurosurgery. 8th edition, 2016, page 775.

123.

B Hemangioma

Hemangiomas of the skull can cause areas of skull protrusion with evidence of trabeculated bone on X-ray. During surgery they appear bluish in color underneath the pericranium. They should be excised completely to avoid recurrence.

Further Reading: Greenberg. Handbook of Neurosurgery. 8th edition, 2016, page 776.

124.

A Diabetes insipidus

The Hand-Schüller-Christian triad is a series of clinical symptoms caused by an underlying diagnosis of Langerhans cell histiocytosis. When this occurs in the suprasellar region, a mass emanating from the pituitary stalk can cause diabetes insipidus.

Further Reading: Greenberg. Handbook of Neurosurgery. 8th edition, 2016, page 777.

125.

C McCune-Albright syndrome

Fibrous dysplasia is a benign condition where bone is replaced by fibrous connective tissue, and it is seen commonly in McCune-Albright syndrome along with endocrine dysfunction, café au lait spots on one side of the midline, and precocious puberty.

Further Reading: Greenberg. Handbook of Neurosurgery. 8th edition, 2016, page 781.

126.

D Needle aspiration of cystic contents

While all of the above options are reasonable to decrease intracranial pressure, when a mass has a large cystic component, simple drainage of the cyst can lead to rapid decompression of the posterior fossa.

127.

B No

Generally, the wall of the associated cyst cavity within a hemangioblastoma does not need to be resected, unless there is a portion that enhances. Removal of the enhancing mural nodule should lead to sufficient resection.

128.

A Yes

Generally, the wall of the associated cyst cavity should be resected if it can be done safely. Certain pilocytic astrocytomas can have pseudocysts that are really more tumor tissue and attempts should be made to resect the wall if possible. Certainly any areas that are enhancing should be resected if it can be done safely.

129.

C Fornix

When the endoscope is advanced through the foramen of Monro, care should be taken to avoid significant manipulation if possible given that the fornix can be easily compressed on the superior aspect of the foramen by a rigid endoscope.

Further Reading: Torres-Corzo, Rangel-Castilla, Nakaji. Neuroendoscopic Surgery, 2016, page 232.

130.

B 3 to 4.5 cm

Approximately 3 to 4.5 cm of dominant temporal lobe can be resected safely. Further posterior and risk to language function increases.

Further Reading: Baltuch, Villemure. Operative Techniques in Epilepsy Surgery, 2009, page 40.

131.

B 2

The WFNS grade is a way to evaluate clinical symptoms after SAH. A patient with a GCS of 13 to 14 without major motor deficit would be considered a WFNS grade 2.

Further Reading: Greenberg. Handbook of Neurosurgery. 8th edition, 2016, page 1163.

132.

C 33%

The modified Fisher scale rates the amount and location of SAH to predict risk of vasospasm. Grade 1 is thin (< 3 mm) clot only with no IVH–24% risk. Grade 2 is thin (< 3 mm) clot with IVH–33% RISK. Grade 3 is thick (> 3 mm) clot with no IVH–33% risk, and grade 4 is thick clot with IVH–40% risk.

Further Reading: Spetzler, Kalani, Nakaji. Neurovascular Surgery, 2nd edition, 2015, page 471.

133.

A 1.5%

After aneurysmal rupture there is an approximately 1.5% per day risk of rebleeding up to 13 days postbleed. At 6 months there is a risk of 50%.

Further Reading: Greenberg. Handbook of Neurosurgery. 8th edition, 2016, page 1168.

134.

C Vasospasm

This patient is likely experiencing a vasospasm, which occurs usually between postbleed days 3 and 14. It is rare for vasospasm to occur < 3 days.

Further Reading: Greenberg. Handbook of Neurosurgery. 8th edition, 2016, page 1178.

135.

A Anterior communicating artery

Anterior communicating artery aneurysms are the most common location for intracranial aneurysms (30%).

Further Reading: Greenberg. Handbook of Neurosurgery. 8th edition, 2016, page 1191.

136.

B Posterior communicating artery

Posterior communicating artery aneurysms classically present with a non-pupil sparing third nerve palsy (due to compression and not microvascular disease, which would be pupil sparing). While only 9% of posterior communicating artery aneurysms will present this way, given the location of the posterior communicating artery to the third nerve, it is a commonly tested subject.

Further Reading: Greenberg. Handbook of Neurosurgery. 8th edition, 2016, page 1192.

137.

C Proximal control

Obtaining proximal control prior to dissecting the aneurysm or placing a clip. When proximal control is obtained, further dissection can take place. If the aneurysm ruptures, temporary clips can be applied to the areas of proximal control in order to decrease bleeding.

Further Reading: Spetzler, Kalani, Nakaji. Neurovascular Surgery, 2nd edition, 2015, page 1106.

138.

B Right superior nasal quadrantanopsia

Ophthalmic segment aneurysms can grow and cause compression of the optic nerve. Given that they will compress the nerve from the inferior temporal side, you would expect him to have an ipsilateral superior nasal quadrantanopsia.

Further Reading: Greenberg. Handbook of Neurosurgery. 8th edition, 2016, page 1214.

139.

A Falciform ligament

The falciform ligament is a dural fold overlying the superior aspect of the optic nerve. When an aneurysm pushes the optic nerve superiorly, compression can occur from above as the nerve is pressed against the falciform ligament. After an anterior clinoidectomy, opening of the falciform ligament can decompress the optic nerve.

Further Reading: Greenberg. Handbook of Neurosurgery. 8th edition, 2016, page 1214.

140.

C CT head

Occasionally patients can have bridging bone between the anterior and posterior clinoid processes, so called the "middle clinoid process." If the surgeon is unaware of the presence of this middle clinoid process bridging bone, aggressive removal of the anterior clinoid process can lead to transection of the carotid artery as the bridging bone often encases the carotid artery to some degree. A CT scan of the head can rule out the presence of the middle clinoid bridging bone.

Further Reading: Spetzler, Kalani, Nakaji. Neurovascular Surgery, 2nd edition, 2015, page 17.

141.

B 3

The Spetzler-Martin grading system applies to AVMs and takes into account size of the nidus (< 3 cm, 3–6 cm, > 6 cm), venous drainage (deep/superficial), and location (eloquent/noneloquent cortex). The scale is 1 to 5.

Further Reading: Greenberg. Handbook of Neurosurgery, 8th edition, 2016, page 1243.

142.

B 84%

Based on the Spetzler-Martin grading system, grade 3 AVMs have an 84% chance of good outcome after surgical resection (grade 1 = 100%, grade 2 = 95%, grade 3 = 84%, grade 4 = 73%, grade 5 = 69%).

Further Reading: Greenberg. Handbook of Neurosurgery, 8th edition, 2016, page 1243.

143.

B 3.5%

The approximate annual risk of hemorrhage for grade 1 to 3 AVMs is 3.5%.

Further Reading: Greenberg. Handbook of Neurosurgery, 8th edition, 2016, page 1240.

144.

B False

Many cavernous malformations of the brain are associated with developmental venous anomalies. It is important to remember that these venous channels can drain normal brain tissue and should not be resected to avoid risk of postoperative venous stroke.

Further Reading: Greenberg. Handbook of Neurosurgery, 8th edition, 2016, page 1245.

145.

A True

When cavernous malformations hemorrhage they can cause hemosiderin staining of the surrounding brain parenchyma which gives it a yellowish color. Many surgeons believe that this hemosiderin stained brain can be a seizure focus and should be resected if it can be done safely.

Further Reading: Greenberg. Handbook of Neurosurgery, 8th edition, 2016, page 1250.

146.

D Pulsatile tinnitus

The vast majority of dural arteriovenous fistulae present with pulsatile tinnitus.

Further Reading: Greenberg. Handbook of Neurosurgery, 8th edition, 2016, page 1251.

147.

C Retrograde sinus and retrograde cortical venous drainage

There are two major classification systems for dural arteriovenous fistulae, the Borden classification and the Cognard classification. The Cognard classification consists of type I (anterograde drainage through a sinus), type IIa (retrograde sinus drainage only), type IIb (anterograde sinus drainage with retrograde cortical venous reflux), type II a + b (retrograde sinus and retrograde cortical venous reflux), type III (direct cortical venous drainage without ectasia), type IV (direct cortical venous drainage with ectasia), and type V (direct drainage into spinal perimedullary veins).

Further Reading: Greenberg. Handbook of Neurosurgery, 8th edition, 2016, page 1254.

148.

A Type II a + b

Type II a + b (retrograde sinus and cortical venous reflux) carries the highest risk of hemorrhage, approximately 66%. Next is type IV with direct cortical venous drainage with ectasia, at 65%.

Further Reading: Greenberg. Handbook of Neurosurgery, 8th edition, 2016, page 1254.

149.

C Heart failure

Vein of Galen malformations present in neonates with evidence of high output heart failure.

Further Reading: Greenberg. Handbook of Neurosurgery, 8th edition, 2016, page 1256.

150.

D Carotid-cavernous fistula

Traumatic carotid-cavernous fistulae can occur after motor vehicle accidents or other intracranial trauma. They present with orbital pain, chemosis, proptosis, ophthalmoplegia, and visual loss. Patients should undergo vascular imaging and may require interventional or surgical treatment of the fistula.

Further Reading: Greenberg. Handbook of Neurosurgery, 8th edition, 2016, page 1257.

151.

B False

Radiation therapy damages cells by firing particles into an atom and releasing free electrons causing damage downstream. In fully oxygenated cells, oxygen combines with unpaired free electrons to form peroxides, which are more stable and lethal than free radicals, and therefore an oxygenated cell is more sensitive to damage by radiation therapy.

Further Reading: Greenberg. Handbook of Neurosurgery, 8th edition, 2016, page 1566.

152.

B > 3 years

Children less than 3 years of age are particularly sensitive to cranial radiation and can have severe developmental side effects. Children should be greater than 3 years of age to be eligible for cranial radiation. There may be demonstrable changes in IQ (decrease by 25 points) in children who receive radiation up to 7 years of age.

Further Reading: Keating, Goodrich, Packer. Tumors of the Pediatric Central Nervous System, 2nd edition, 2013, page 138.

153.

B 3 cm or less

Gamma knife radiosurgery can be useful for cranial masses, but should be reserved for patients with brain tumors that are 3 cm or less in maximum diameter. This size cutoff decreases the risk of harmful radiation side effects to surrounding brain structures.

Further Reading: Greenberg. Handbook of Neurosurgery. 8th edition, 2016, page 1564.

154.

B 10 Gy

Safe doses of radiation to the optic apparatus are generally thought to be 8 to 10 Gy. Doses beyond this can lead to visual loss.

Further Reading: Greenberg. Handbook of Neurosurgery. 8th edition, 2016, page 1567.

Lunsford, Sheehan. Intracranial Stereotactic Radiosurgery, 2016, page 52.

155.

B 13 Gy or less

SRS doses for vestibular schwannomas have changed based on recent literature, and currently 12 to 13 Gy to the facial nerve seems to be a dose of radiation that causes good tumor control but greatly decreases the side effects to the seventh and eighth nerve.

Further Reading: Lunsford, Sheehan. Intracranial Stereotactic Radiosurgery, 2016, page 150.

156.

C 10 Gy or less

The lens of the eye can tolerate 10 Gy or less radiation with minimal side effects. Cataract formation will occur with doses up to 50 Gy.

Further Reading: Greenberg. Handbook of Neurosurgery. 8th edition, 2016, page 1567

Lunsford, Sheehan. Intracranial Stereotactic Radiosurgery, 2016, page 52.

157.

D 40 to 50%

At 10 years posttreatment, approximately 40 to 50% of patients who receive sellar radiation will experience hypopituitarism as a side effect from radiation.

Further Reading: Greenberg. Handbook of Neurosurgery. 8th edition, 2016, page 744.

Lunsford, Sheehan. Intracranial Stereotactic Radiosurgery, 2016, page 107.

158.

B 4 to 6 Gy

Based on current literature, the mean safe radiation dose to the cochlea is considered to be approximately 4.2 Gy, but has also been shown to range from 4 to 6 Gy. There is some controversy on this topic currently, but based on data available, doses from 4 to 6 Gy should be considered optimal.

Further Reading: Greenberg. Handbook of Neurosurgery. 8th edition, 2016, page 1570.

Lunsford, Sheehan Intracranial Stereotactic Radiosurgery, 2016, page 52.

159.

C 24 Gy

For tumors that are 10 to 20 mm, SRS doses up to 24 Gy can be used with acceptable risk of side effects.

Further Reading: Greenberg. Handbook of Neurosurgery. 8th edition, 2016, page 1570.

Lunsford, Sheehan. Intracranial Stereotactic Radiosurgery, 2016, page 235.

160.

B 18 Gy

For tumors that are 21 to 30 mm, SRS doses up to 18 Gy can be used with acceptable risk of side effects.

Further Reading: Greenberg. Handbook of Neurosurgery. 8th edition, 2016, page 1570.

Lunsford, Sheehan. Intracranial Stereotactic Radiosurgery, 2016, page 235.

161.

C Whole brain radiation

Current literature supports the use of whole brain radiation in patients who have undergone resection of a cerebral metastasis. Doses up to 50 Gy have been shown to control > 90% of micrometasases, but at this dose there is a very high chance of early radiation side effects.

Further Reading: Greenberg. Handbook of Neurosurgery. 8th edition, 2016, page 808.

162.

B 10 or less

Based on current studies, up to 10 concurrent cerebral metastases can be treated with stereotactic radiosurgery with good outcome and low risk of side effects. There are surgeons who feel that even this number can be safely extended, research is pending.

Further Reading: Greenberg. Handbook of Neurosurgery. 8th edition, 2016, page 1568.

Lunsford, Sheehan. Intracranial Stereotactic Radiosurgery, 2016, page 243.

163.

D < 3 years

Stereotactic radiosurgery can be a good option for low grade AVMs with a well formed nidus that border eloquent cortex. Radiation works by causing damage to the endothelium and ultimately causing fibrosis. This process can take 2 to 3 years to develop, so risk of hemorrhage needs to be discussed with the patient over that treatment timeframe.

Further Reading: Greenberg. Handbook of Neurosurgery. 8th edition, 2016, page 1568.

Lunsford, Sheehan. Intracranial Stereotactic Radiosurgery, 2016, page 68.

164.

C 23 to 25 Gy

Current literature suggests that 23 to 25 Gy radiation doses to AVMs lead to high rates of obliteration with low risk of complications. Higher radiation doses have been associated with an increased risk of complications and no significant improvement in obliteration rates.

Further Reading: Greenberg. Handbook of Neurosurgery. 8th edition, 2016, page 1568.

Lunsford, Sheehan. Intracranial Stereotactic Radiosurgery, 2016, page 68.

165.

D 70 to 80%

Current literature suggests that 70 to 80% of all AVMs treated with stereotactic radiosurgery may achieve complete obliteration by 2 to 3 years after treatment.

Further Reading: Greenberg. Handbook of Neurosurgery. 8th edition, 2016, page 1568.

166.

C 65%

While up to 86% of patients will experience a decrease in their pain after SRS for TGN, the long term pain free rate is approximately 65%.

Further Reading: Greenberg. Handbook of Neurosurgery. 8th edition, 2016, page 485.

Lunsford, Sheehan. Intracranial Stereotactic Radiosurgery, 2016, page 160.

167.

D Dementia

Dementia is the main complication from whole brain radiation after use for intracranial metastases. Symptoms can develop as quickly as 1 year

after WBRT is performed. Incidence has been shown to be higher when patients receiving doses of 25 to 39 Gy receive those doses in fractionations that are > 300c Gy

Further Reading: Greenberg. Handbook of Neurosurgery. 8th edition, 2016, page 1561.

Lunsford, Sheehan. Intracranial Stereotactic Radiosurgery, 2016, page 52.

168.

A 8 Gy

Emergency radiation can be delivered to radiosensitive spine tumors when there is evidence of compression. In many circumstances, an initial dose of 8 Gy will be given to shrink the tumor, followed by further fractionated radiation after the acute situation has resolved.

Further Reading: Greenberg. Handbook of Neurosurgery. 8th edition, 2016, page 1562.

169.

C 30 Gy in 10 fractions

Radiation to the spine for metastatic disease in the setting of radiosensitive tumors is often administered at a dose of 30 Gy delivered over 10 fractions.

Further Reading: Greenberg. Handbook of Neurosurgery. 8th edition, 2016, page 1562.

170.

C 75%

While TGN can be treated medically, approximately 75% of patients will require a procedure directed at treating the TGN.

Further Reading: Greenberg. Handbook of Neurosurgery. 8th edition, 2016, page 479.

171.

A Anesthesia dolorosa

Anesthesia dolorosa is a feared complication of intentional damage to the trigeminal nerve. It occurs after damage to the V1 segment of the nerve, and can lead to anesthesia of the cornea, causing patients to get recurrent corneal abrasions. Significant care should be taken to avoid injuring the V1 segment.

Further Reading: Greenberg. Handbook of Neurosurgery. 8th edition, 2016, page 479.

172.

B MRI brain with FIESTA sequences

This patient appears to have symptoms consistent with trigeminal neuralgia. Initially, imaging of the brain should be performed to rule out mass lesions or evidence of multiple sclerosis.

Further Reading: Greenberg. Handbook of Neurosurgery. 8th edition, 2016, page 479.

173.

A Start carbamazepine

This patient appears to have symptoms consistent with trigeminal neuralgia. Initially, imaging of the brain should be performed to rule out mass lesions or evidence of multiple sclerosis. Following this, a trial of medical management utilizing carbamazepine 100 mg BID is a reasonable option.

Further Reading: Greenberg. Handbook of Neurosurgery. 8th edition, 2016, page 479.

174.

C 70%

At 10 years, microvascular decompression has a pain free rate of 70%. It is an excellent option for patients who can tolerate a small craniotomy and have a life expectancy of longer than 5 years.

Further Reading: Greenberg. Handbook of Neurosurgery. 8th edition, 2016, page 479.

175.

C Fluid status

SIADH and CSW are both conditions that cause hyponatremia and can be seen after aneurysmal rupture. It is important to determine the difference between the two as treatment is different. CSW causes patients to be hypovolemic whereas in SIADH patients are euvolemic.

Further Reading: Greenberg. Handbook of Neurosurgery. 8th edition, 2016, page 110.

176.

B Fluid restriction

In SIADH, patients are euvolemic or hypervolemic and hyponatremic. In a patient who can tolerate PO intake and is conscious, fluid restriction is a good initial step in management assuming the hyponatremia is not severe.

Further Reading: Greenberg. Handbook of Neurosurgery. 8th edition, 2016, page 118.

177.

D Demeclocycline

Demeclocycline is a tetracycline antibiotic that has side effects including antagonism of ADH. It can be used for medical management of SIADH if fluid restriction is not normalizing the sodium.

Further Reading: Greenberg. Handbook of Neurosurgery. 8th edition, 2016, page 118.

178.

B Fludrocortisone

Fludrocortisone acts directly on renal tubules to increase sodium absorption and can be a useful medication adjunct when treating cerebral salt wasting.

Further Reading: Greenberg. Handbook of Neurosurgery. 8th edition, 2016, page 119.

179.

A Normal saline infusion

In cerebral salt wasting, patients are hypovolemic and hyponatremic. Fluid resuscitation with normal saline at 100 to 125 mL/hr should be instituted in an attempt to normalize fluid status.

Further Reading: Greenberg. Handbook of Neurosurgery. 8th edition, 2016, page 119.

180.

B Severe dehydration

The main complication of untreated diabetes insipidus is severe dehydration

Further Reading: Greenberg. Handbook of Neurosurgery. 8th edition, 2016, page 120.

181.

C 85%

Approximately 85% capacity to secrete ADH must be lost before symptoms of DI will be evident.

Further Reading: Greenberg. Handbook of Neurosurgery. 8th edition, 2016, page 120.

182.

A Drink to thirst

In an awake, conscious and ambulatory patient with mild diabetes insipidus, sodium levels should be monitored, but patients should be allowed to drink to thirst. They are often able to effectively manage their sodium via thirst mechanisms. Utilization of DDAVP occurs in unconscious patients or those who cannot adequately compensate using standard thirst mechanisms.

Further Reading: Greenberg. Handbook of Neurosurgery. 8th edition, 2016, page 123.

183.

C > 10 µg/kg/min

At doses from 2-10 µg/kg/min, dopamine is a positive inotrope, but remember that at least 25% of IV dopamine is converted to norepinephrine, so at doses > 10 µg/kg/min you are essentially giving norepinephrine and the alpha/beta/dopaminergic receptors are all activated.

Further Reading: Greenberg. Handbook of Neurosurgery. 8th edition, 2016, page 128.

184.

D 72 hours

Dobutamine increases cardiac output by positive inotropy, but patients will exhibit tachyphylaxis after approximately 72 hours of administration.

Further Reading: Greenberg. Handbook of Neurosurgery. 8th edition, 2016, page 128.

185.

C < 3 weeks

Generally speaking, patients who are on daily steroid medications should receive GI prophylaxis to prevent steroid induced ulcers after they have been on the medication for 3 weeks or longer. Acutely hospitalized patients or postoperative patients on steroids should be on GI prophylaxis as the stress of the hospitalization can lead to stress ulcer formation

Further Reading: Greenberg. Handbook of Neurosurgery. 8th edition, 2016, page 129.

186.

B 5 to 10K

One unit of platelets (out of the standard six pack) will raise the platelet count approximately 5 to 10K.

Further Reading: Greenberg. Handbook of Neurosurgery. 8th edition, 2016, page 155.

187.

A 10K

In the absence of evidence of bleeding, platelets should be transfused prophylactically when the count drops to 10K.

Further Reading: Greenberg. Handbook of Neurosurgery. 8th edition, 2016, page 154.

188.

B 1 mg protamine/100 u heparin

Protamine sulfate can be used to reverse the effects of unfractionated heparin, and should be administered in doses of 1 mg protamine/100 u heparin.

Further Reading: Greenberg. Handbook of Neurosurgery. 8th edition, 2016, page 158.

189.

B 4 hours

Idarucizumab (Praxbind) is an effective reversal agent for the direct thrombin inhibitor Dabigatran (Pradaxa). It reverses the effects within 4 hours and lasts for 24 hours.

Further Reading: Greenberg. Handbook of Neurosurgery. 8th edition, 2016, page 165.

190.

C Malignant hyperthermia

Malignant hyperthermia can occur after anesthetic use of volatile anesthetics, specifically halothane, or muscle relaxants such as succinylcholine. It is characterized by rigidity, tachycardia, tachypnea and severe fever.

Further Reading: Keating, Goodrich, Packer. Tumors of the Pediatric Central Nervous System, 2nd edition, 2013, page 131.

191.

C Dantrolene

Malignant hyperthermia can occur after anesthetic use of volatile anesthetics, specifically halothane, or muscle relaxants such as succinylcholine. It is characterized by rigidity, tachycardia, tachypnea and severe fever. It should be treated with administration of dantrolene.

Further Reading: Keating, Goodrich, Packer. Tumors of the Pediatric Central Nervous System, 2nd edition, 2013, page 131.

192.

B Ryanodine

Malignant hyperthermia can occur after anesthetic use of volatile anesthetics, specifically halothane, or muscle relaxants such as succinylcholine. It is characterized by rigidity, tachycardia, tachypnea and severe fever. It should be treated with administration of dantrolene. It is thought to occur in some cases due to genetic defects in the ryanodine receptor on the sarcoplasmic reticulum.

Further Reading: Keating, Goodrich, Packer. Tumors of the Pediatric Central Nervous System, 2nd edition, 2013, page 131.

193.

C 17%

Based on NASCET, in patients with symptomatic high grade stenosis who undergo CEA with an acceptable perioperative risk, the reduction in stroke rate is 17% at 18 months.

Further Reading: Greenberg. Handbook of Neurosurgery. 8th edition, 2016, page 1290.

Harbaugh, Shaffrey, Couldwell, Berger. Neurosurgery Knowledge Update, 2015, page 96.

194.

B 3% or less

Current literature suggests that you should have a 3% or less overall complication rate to justify performing a carotid endarterectomy.

Further Reading: Greenberg. Handbook of Neurosurgery, 8th edition, 2016, page 1292.

Harbaugh, Shaffrey, Couldwell, Berger. Neurosurgery Knowledge Update, 2015, page 96.

195.

B CT angiogram

This patient is experiencing return of her preoperative symptoms after CEA. It is possible that the CEA site is undergoing thrombosis and should be emergently evaluated with a CT angiogram to determine patency of the vessel. If occluded, she should return to the OR for re-opening and treatment of the occlusion.

Further Reading: Greenberg. Handbook of Neurosurgery, 8th edition, 2016, page 1293.

Harbaugh, Shaffrey, Couldwell, Berger. Neurosurgery Knowledge Update, 2015, page 96.

196.

C Blood pressure control

This patient is likely experiencing cerebral hyperperfusion syndrome given that blood flow to the ipsilateral hemisphere has now greatly increased. This is a controversial area, but close blood pressure control can help decrease the symptoms of cerebral hyperperfusion syndrome. Imaging should be obtained as well to ensure that no hemorrhage has occurred.

Further Reading: Greenberg. Handbook of Neurosurgery, 8th edition, 2016, page 1293.

Harbaugh, Shaffrey, Couldwell, Berger. Neurosurgery Knowledge Update, 2015, page 96.

197.

A Hypoglossal palsy

The distal hypoglossal nerve is often seen during the dissection for a carotid endarterectomy and a postoperative palsy has been reported to be as high as 8% in some series. Care should be taken to avoid damaging the hypoglossal nerve during the dissection.

Further Reading: Greenberg. Handbook of Neurosurgery, 8th edition, 2016, page 1293.

Harbaugh, Shaffrey, Couldwell, Berger. Neurosurgery Knowledge Update, 2015, page 96.

198.

B Bedside decompression

This patient has an obvious arteriotomy closure disruption and it is causing tracheal deviation and respiratory compromise. While you may think intubation would be the initial management option, it can be difficult or impossible in patients with severe tracheal deviation, so bedside decompression of the clot should occur immediately, followed by intubation and return to the OR.

Further Reading: Greenberg. Handbook of Neurosurgery, 8th edition, 2016, page 1294.

199.

B 2 weeks

Pooled analysis of the symptomatic carotid stenosis trials have demonstrated that there is a benefit for patients who receive a CEA within 2 weeks of stroke compared to those patients who had a CEA at greater than 2 weeks.

Further Reading: Greenberg. Handbook of Neurosurgery, 8th edition, 2016, page 1291.

Harbaugh, Shaffrey, Couldwell, Berger. Neurosurgery Knowledge Update, 2015, page 96.

200.

D Noninferiority

The CREST trial demonstrated non-inferiority of carotid angioplasty and stenting to open carotid endarterectomy. In many practices, surgeons utilize carotid angioplasty and stenting in patients with high-riding carotid bifurcations or very difficult appearing stenosis that might have a higher rate of operative complications.

Further Reading: Harbaugh, Shaffrey, Couldwell, Berger. Neurosurgery Knowledge Update, 2015, page 96.

9 Neurology

1.

B Aquaporin channel

This patient has neuromyelitis optica (Devic's disease) which is a variant of multiple sclerosis that involves the optic nerves and often presents with longitudinal spinal cord T2 signal change that spans three levels (compared with transverse myelitis which does not span that many segments).

Further Reading: Borsody. Comprehensive Board Review in Neurology, 2007, page 110.

2.

D JC virus infection

This patient has classic signs and symptoms of progressive multifocal leukoencephalopathy, caused by JC virus infection that destroys oligodendrocytes in patients with AIDS. It often presents as an asymmetric, parieto-occipital area of demyelination.

Further Reading: Borsody. Comprehensive Board Review in Neurology, 2007, page 259.

Forsting, Jansen. MR Neuroimaging: Brain, Spine, Peripheral Nerves, 2017, page 184.

3.

B Botulism

Both myasthenia gravis and botulism can affect extraocular muscles but the pupils are spared in myasthenia and involved in botulism.

Further Reading: Borsody. Comprehensive Board Review in Neurology, 2007, page 235.

4.

C Dorsal midbrain

This patient has convergence-retraction nystagmus, which can be a form of Perinaud's syndrome, caused by compression or destruction of dorsal midbrain nuclei.

Further Reading: Alberstone, Benzel, Najm, Steinmetz. Anatomic Basis of Neurologic Diagnosis, 2009, page 453.

5.

D Miosis

Pontine hemorrhage leads to bilateral pinpoint pupils. This occurs because the descending sympathetic tracts are disrupted while the parasympathetic tracts to the pupil remain intact.

Further Reading: Alberstone, Benzel, Najm, Steinmetz. Anatomic Basis of Neurologic Diagnosis, 2009, pages 502–503.

6.

C Third order neuron

The third order neuron involved in pupillary dilation must be intact for Paredrine to cause dilation of the pupil.

Further Reading: Laws, Sheehan. Sellar and Parasellar Tumors, 2012, page 99.

7.

A Autosomal recessive

Friedrich's ataxia is caused by a mutation in the frataxin gene, and dysfunction causes failure of iron transport into mitochondria. It often involves a trinucleotide repeat and causes degeneration of the dentate nucleus and spinocerebellar tract. It is inherited in an autosomal recessive fashion.

Further Reading: Borsody. Comprehensive Board Review in Neurology, 2007, page 199.

8.

A Neurofibromatosis type I

Sphenoid hypoplasia is often seen in patients with NF1.

Further Reading: Harbaugh, Shaffrey, Couldwell, Berger. Neurosurgery Knowledge Update, 2015, page 431.

9.

B Epstein-Barr virus/B cell type

Lymphoma is thought to develop in up to 5% of patients with HIV. It is associated with Epstein-Barr virus. It is a B cell lymphoma. Treatment involves chemotherapy and dexamethasone as well as whole brain radiation. Survival is short, with the median survival being 3 months.

Further Reading: Siddiqi. Neurosurgical Intensive Care, 2017, page 376.

10.

C Tau protein

Neurofibrillary tangles are found in patients with Alzheimer's dementia. They are comprised of tau protein.

Further Reading: Borsody. Comprehensive Board Review in Neurology, 2007, page 156.

11.

D Occipital cortex

Alzheimer's dementia is graded pathologically, and when neurofibrillary tangles and plaques are found in the occipital cortex, the highest grade (grade IV disease) is diagnosed.

Further Reading: Borsody. Comprehensive Board Review in Neurology, 2007, page 155.

12.

C Dystrophin/completely absent

This describes a patient with Duchenne's muscular dystrophy, a rapidly progressive muscular dystrophy causing wasting of proximal muscles. It is caused in many cases by a frameshift mutation which leads to complete absence of the dystrophin gene. Becker's muscle dystrophy causes partial dysfunction of the dystrophin gene but has similar symptoms to Duchenne's, except that it progresses in a much slower fashion.

Further Reading: Borsody. Comprehensive Board Review in Neurology, 2007, page 238.

13.

E Anti-Ma

Patients with limbic encephalitis can be found to have autoantibodies (Anti-Ma). It is important to rule out herpes encephalitis in these patients.

Further Reading: Citow, Macdonald, Refai. Comprehensive Neurosurgery Board Review, 2nd edition, 2010, page 223.

14.

C ATP pump failure

The cognitive dysfunction that occurs in the postconcussive syndrome is thought to occur due to ATP pump failure at the cellular level. There are multiple cellular events that are also thought to be associated with this condition.

Further Reading: Harbaugh, Shaffrey, Couldwell, Berger. Neurosurgery Knowledge Update, 2015, page 757.

15.

B Cognitive rest

Patients who have experienced a concussion should go through a regimen of cognitive and physical rest until they can progress through stages of increased activity without symptoms.

Further Reading: Harbaugh, Shaffrey, Couldwell, Berger. Neurosurgery Knowledge Update, 2015, page 759.

16.

B Functional hemispherectomy

Rasmussen's encephalitis is a debilitating disease process that causes epilepsy partialis continua in some patients. Prolonged seizures lead to intellectual disability and significant brain dysfunction. Functional hemispherectomy has been utilized to treat this condition.

Further Reading: Albright, Pollack, Adelson. Principles and Practice of Pediatric Neurosurgery, 3rd edition, 2015, page 986.

17.

C Ethosuxamide

This EEG demonstrates a burst of generalized 3 Hz spike and wave activity associated with absence seizures. These seizures are best treated with ethosuxamide.

Further Reading: Borsody. Comprehensive Board Review in Neurology, 2007, page 95.

18.

A < 5%

In patients who experience a simple febrile seizure, very few (< 5%) will go on to develop any ongoing epilepsy after the initial febrile seizure.

Further Reading: Borsody. Comprehensive Board Review in Neurology, 2007, page 91.

19.

C Joubert syndrome

This MRI demonstrates the "molar tooth" malformation commonly seen in Joubert syndrome. There is cerebellar peduncle hypoplasia, a small midbrain and a batwing-shaped fourth ventricle.

Further Reading: Forsting, Jansen. MR Neuroimaging: Brain, Spine, Peripheral Nerves, 2017, page 316.

20.

A Pain before weakness

Brachial neuritis can occur after viral infection, and sometimes in the postoperative setting. The full pathophysiology is not well understood, but is thought to be an inflammatory reaction in multiple nerve distributions. It presents with severe shoulder pain followed by resolution and then development of motor weakness of the affected extremity.

Further Reading: Mackinnon, Yee. Nerve Surgery, 2015, page 403.

21.

C Blue rubber bleb nevus syndrome

This patient has a persistent connection between the extracranial veins and the superior sagittal sinus, known as sinus pericranii. This is often seen in patients with blue rubber bleb nevus syndrome.

Further Reading: Meyers. Differential Diagnosis in Neuroimaging: Head and Neck, 2017, page 43.

22.

B Arsenic

Mees' transverse white lines on the fingernails are associated with arsenic exposure.

Further Reading: Citow, Macdonald, Refai. Comprehensive Neurosurgery Board Review, 2nd edition, 2010, page 296.

23.

A Dysembryoplastic gangliocytoma of the cerebellum

Dysembryoplastic gangliocytoma of the cerebellum (Lhermitte-Duclos disease) is a finding associated with PTEN mutations and Cowden's syndrome. This syndrome is also associated with multiple trichilemmomas, breast, and endometrial carcinoma.

Further Reading: Bernstein, Berger. Neuro-Oncology: The Essentials, 3rd edition, 2015, page 309.

24.

C REM sleep

Patients with narcolepsy exhibit sleep-onset REM. This is classic for this condition.

Further Reading: Borsody. Comprehensive Board Review in Neurology, 2007, page 167.

25.

B F2

EEG electrodes are placed in a standard fashion, with corresponding letters as follows: F = frontal, C = central, P = parietal, O = occipital. Even numbers correspond with the right side of the head, and odd numbers correspond to the left side of the head.

Further Reading: Blume WT, Buza RC, Okazaki H. Anatomic correlates of the ten-twenty electrode placement system in infants. Electroencephalogr Clin Neurophysiol 1974; 36(3):303–307.

http://faculty.washington.edu/chudler/1020.html

26.

D Bithalamic destruction

While respiratory patterns are difficult and unreliable for diagnosing lesion locations, Cheyne-Stokes respiratory patterns (waxing and waning respiratory patterns) can be seen in patients with bithalamic injury.

Further Reading: Rohkamm. Color Atlas of Neurology, 2007, page 118.

27.

A Pituitary adenoma enlargement

Nelson's syndrome occurs when a patient with a previously unknown ACTH secreting pituitary adenoma undergoes a bilateral adrenalectomy. Loss of feedback inhibition of ACTH production leads to rapid enlargement of the pituitary adenoma.

Further Reading: Gasco, Nader. The Essential Neurosurgery Companion, 2013, page 533.

28.

A Low serum ceruloplasmin, high urine copper

This image demonstrates Kayser-Fleischer rings and confirms the diagnosis of Wilson's disease. This patient would be expected to have low serum ceruloplasmin and high urinary excretion of copper.

Further Reading: Borsody. Comprehensive Board Review in Neurology, 2007, page 195.

29.

B Positioning-related brachial plexus compression

Erb's point is near the shoulder and when sensory latency is prolonged at Erb's point, a positioning palsy of the brachial plexus should be considered. In this case, with a low ACDF, pulling on the shoulders to achieve a better X-ray line of sight can lead to brachial plexus traction.

Further Reading: Newton, O'Brien, Shufflebarger, Betz, Dickson, Harms. Idiopathic Scoliosis, 2011, page 373.

30.

B Painful and temporary

Diabetic third nerve palsies are often pupil-sparing (center of the nerve is involved rather than the parasympathetic fibers that travel in the peripheral aspect of the nerve). It is painful and temporary.

Further Reading: Borsody. Comprehensive Board Review in Neurology, 2007, page 43.

31.

D Sympathetic blockade

This patient has complex regional pain syndrome type I (no nerve injury). Often medications are used to treat this condition, but when these fail, sympathetic blockade can be considered. Neurectomy and cordotomy may worsen the condition.

Further Reading: Harbaugh, Shaffrey, Couldwell, Berger. Neurosurgery Knowledge Update, 2015, page 740.

32.

C Homocystinuria

This patient has a transverse sinus thrombosis which has resulted in a temporal lobe infarction. Patients with homocystinuria can have prothrombotic states that lead to intracranial sinus thrombosis.

Further Reading: Kanekar. Imaging of Neurodegenerative Disorders, 2016, page 213.

33.

C 48 hours

Pentobarbital is a long-acting sedative that can be used for refractory ICP elevation. When therapy is ceased, it can take 48 hours for neurologic function to return.

Further Reading: Siddiqi. Neurosurgical Intensive Care, 2017, page 162.

34.

C Dorsal root ganglion

The H-reflex is used in the S1 nerve and approximates the reflex arc of the spinal cord. Signal is sent through the peripheral sensory nerves and motor response is recorded. The F-wave involves supramaximal stimulation of the peripheral motor nerves and the wave propagates proximally through the nerve root into the spinal canal, also firing several other nerve roots as well in the process. It is a way to determine the integrity of the motor roots. If the H-reflex is absent but the F-wave is normal, the problem is likely to be in the DRG.

Further Reading: Fehlings, Boakye, Ditunno, Vaccaro, Rossignol, Burns. Essentials of Spinal Cord Injury, 2013, page 449.

35.

C Ear vesicles

Ramsay Hunt syndrome (zoster oticus) can present similar to Bell's palsy with facial weakness, but attention should be paid to the development of vesicular rashes on the ear, as this leads to the diagnosis of zoster oticus.

Further Reading: Di Ieva, Lee, Cusimano. Handbook of Skull Base Surgery, 2016, page 194.

36.

D Brain MRI

This patient has vertigo and there are several signs that would make you think this is central in origin rather than peripheral. She is having difficulty standing and walking, it was a fairly acute onset, there is little nausea, and she has both skew deviation and spontaneous direction changing nystagmus. MRI will likely demonstrate a cerebellar stroke.

Further Reading: Adunka, Buchman. Otology, Neurotology, and Lateral Skull Base Surgery: An Illustrated Handbook, 2011, page 70.

37.

B Inner hair cells

The inner hair cells of the ear are extremely sensitive to high volume and repeated exposure to high volume can lead to loss of inner hair cells.

Further Reading: Greenstein. Greenstein Color Atlas of Neuroscience, 2000, page 258.

38.

A Medial longitudinal fasciculus

Internuclear ophthalmoplegia can be seen in patients with MS. It is caused by disruption of the medial longitudinal fasciculus, which connects the abducens nucleus to the contralateral oculomotor nucleus in order to preserve conjugate eye movements.

Further Reading: Alberstone, Benzel, Najm, Steinmetz. Anatomic Basis of Neurologic Diagnosis, 2009, page 225.

39.

C Mononeuropathy multiplex

Involvement of multiple, distinct nerves is considered a mononeuropathy multiplex.

Further Reading: Rohkamm. Color Atlas of Neurology, 2007, Page 316.

40.

B Incremental response

Lambert-Eaton syndrome involves autoantibodies directed against calcium channels on the presynaptic membrane. This decreases neurotransmitter release due to lack of calcium. EMG will initially be flat, but with repetitive actions there will be an incremental response as calcium levels increase.

Further Reading: Borsody. Comprehensive Board Review in Neurology, 2007, page 237.

41.

D Toxoplasmosis

This MRI demonstrates classic signs of toxoplasmosis. Toxo is the most common mass lesion in patients with known AIDS.

Further Reading: Hall, Kim. Neurosurgical Infectious Disease, 2014, page 255.

42.

C Leukoencephalopathy

The most common neurological complication of HIV infection is HIV leukoencephalopathy.

Further Reading: Kanekar. Imaging of Neurodegenerative Disorders, 2016, page 22.

43.

B Peripheral neuropathy

Charcot joints (neuropathic osteoarthropathy) are commonly seen in patients with diabetes who have peripheral neuropathy. The neuropathy leads to destruction of the joint over time.

Further Reading: Borsody. Comprehensive Board Review in Neurology, 2007, Page 293.

44.

C Neuroblastoma

Opsoclonus-myoclonus syndrome is a rare disease seen in some patients with neuroblastoma. It is thought to be mediated by an autoimmune phenomenon.

Further Reading: Borsody. Comprehensive Board Review in Neurology, 2007, page 136.

45.

B Corpus callosotomy

Corpus callosotomy is a palliative surgical procedure in patients with intractable drop attacks. It can significantly decrease the frequency of drop attacks in these patients.

Further Reading: Harbaugh, Shaffrey, Couldwell, Berger. Neurosurgery Knowledge Update, 2015, page 409.

46.

A X-linked

This child has Menkes kinky hair syndrome which is a deficiency of copper transport and metabolism, causing copper deficiency. It is inherited in an X-linked fashion. Patients develop subdural hematomas and are found to have tortuous vasculature.

Further Reading: Choudhri. Pediatric Neuroradiology: Clinical Practice Essentials, 2017, page 121.

47.

C Burned in images when eyes are closed

Palinopsia refers to visual preservation, or burned in images when the eyes are closed.

Further Reading: Tsementzis. Differential Diagnosis in Neurology and Neurosurgery, 2000, page 169.

48.

E Tuberous sclerosis

This image demonstrates ungula fibromas, which can be seen in patients with tuberous sclerosis.

Further Reading: Borsody. Comprehensive Board Review in Neurology, 2007, page 277.

49.

B Rosenthal fibers

Alexander disease is a leukodystrophy that can cause significant deficits in infants. It involves a defect of GFAP and on pathologic specimen Rosenthal fibers are commonly seen.

Further Reading: Forsting, Jansen. MR Neuroimaging: Brain, Spine, Peripheral Nerves, 2017, page 250.

50.

D Aphasia

Wernicke's encephalopathy can occur in patients with severe thiamine deficiency and the classic triad includes ataxia, ophthalmoplegia, and confusion. Aphasia is not a component of the triad.

Further Reading: Rohkamm. Color Atlas of Neurology, 2007, page 312.

10 Neuroanatomy

1.

B P2

Ascending deep to the rest of the PCA, the medial posterior choroidal artery supplies the tegmentum, midbrain, posterior thalamus and pineal gland as the cisternal segment. It then penetrates the velum interpositum, running in the roof of the third ventricle supplying the choroid plexus.

Further Reading: Greenberg. Handbook of Neurosurgery, 8th edition, 2016, vascular anatomy section.

2.

C Trochlear

Structures passing through the ambient cistern include the posterior cerebral artery, the supracerebellar artery, the basal veins of Rosenthal and the trochlear nerve (CN IV).

Further Reading: Binder, Sonne, Fischbein. Cranial Nerves: Anatomy, Pathology, Imaging, 2010, chapter 4, trochlear nerve.

3.

D Petrous

The vidian artery originates from the C2 segment of the ICA, the petrous segment. It passes through the vidian canal and can anastamose with a branch of the internal maxillary artery forming an ICA/ECA anastamosis site. The other branch from the C2 (petrous segment) is the caroticotympanic artery.

Further Reading: Greenberg. Handbook of Neurosurgery, 8th edition, 2016, vascular anatomy section.

4.

A Crista galli

The crista galli is a structure arising from the surface of the ethmoid bone, serving as the point of attachment for the falx. It is a midline structure and projects into the anterior cranial fossa.

Further Reading: Wanibuchi, Friedman, Fukushima. Photo Atlas of Skull Base Dissection, 2009, bifrontal transbasal approach.

5.

C Calcarine artery

Brodmann area 17 is the primary visual cortex (V1), also known as the calcarine cortex, and it is the primary input of signals coming from the retina. This cortical region lies inferior to the calcarine sulcus in the medial border of the occipital lobe.

Further Reading: Greenberg. Handbook of Neurosurgery, 8th edition, 2016, vascular anatomy section.

6.

B Inferior frontal gyrus

Brodmann area 44 corresponds to the inferior frontal gyrus, or Broca's area. It is made of three structures, from anterior to posterior, the pars orbitalis, the pars triangularis and the pars opercularis. Broca's area is thought to be formed mainly by the pars triangularis and the pars opercularis.

Further Reading: Greenberg. Handbook of Neurosurgery. 8th edition, 2016, gross anatomy cranial and spine.

7.

B Putamen and globus pallidus

The lentiform nucleus is the combination of the putamen and globus pallidus. Lentiform nucleus comes from lenticular, meaning biconvex, similar to a lens. These structures appear lens-like, giving them this name.

Further Reading: Greenberg. Handbook of Neurosurgery, 8th edition. 2016, gross anatomy cranial and spine.

8.

D External capsule and extreme capsule

The claustrum is a thin sheet of neurons separating the external capsule from the extreme capsule. It receives input from almost all regions of cortex and projects back to almost all regions of cortex. While exact function is not fully understood, it is currently thought to play a role in communication between cerebral hemispheres, and may play a role in attention.

Further Reading: Greenberg. Handbook of Neurosurgery, 8th edition, 2016, gross anatomy cranial and spine.

9.

A Arcuate fasciculus

The arcuate fasciculus is a set of association fibers connecting the superior temporal gyrus/angular gyrus (Wernicke's region) to the inferior frontal gyrus (Broca's area). Lesions disrupting these fibers lead to a conductive aphasia, whereby patients have difficulty repeating phrases, but productive and receptive language remains intact.

Further Reading: Greenberg. Handbook of Neurosurgery, 8th edition, 2016, gross anatomy cranial and spine.

10.

D Ipsilateral monocular blindness

The anterior choroidal artery arises from the internal carotid in the communicating segment (C7). It arises approximately 3 mm distal to the posterior communicating artery and 3 mm proximal from the ICA terminus. It has a characteristic superior bend as it crosses the tentorial edge. Anterior choroidal artery infarctions lead to a characteristic syndrome including contralateral hemiparesis, contralateral hemianesthesia and contralateral hemianiopia. Since the lesion is posterior to the optic chiasm, monocular blindness is not a part of the anterior choroidal artery syndrome.

Further Reading: Greenberg. Handbook of Neurosurgery, 8th edition,. 2016, vascular anatomy section.

11.

B Day 24

The lamina terminalis lies just posterior to the optic chiasm and may be perforated during exposure to drain CSF from the third ventricle and relax the brain. The lamina terminalis is formed after closure of the anterior neuropore on day 24 of development. The posterior neuropore closes on day 26, and forms the neural elements of the lumbar spine.

Further Reading: Torres-Corzo, Rangel-Castilla, Nakaji. Neuroendoscopic Surgery, 2016, lamina terminalis fenestration.

12.

D Ventral posterolateral nuclei–Somatosensory cortex

The thalamus is comprised of multiple relay nuclei and their afferent/efferent projections are often tested on the written boards. The anterior nuclei receive input from the mammillothalamic tract and fornix and project largely to the cingulate cortex. The mediodorsal nuclei receive input from the amygdala, substantia nigra pars reticulata, hippocampus, hypothalamus and entire prefrontal cortex. They project to the orbital frontal cortex and frontal eye fields The VPL nuclei are the primary sensory relay station, they receive input from the medial lemniscus and both spinothalamic tracts (anterior and lateral). The VPL nuclei project to the somatosensory cortex. The pulvinar receives input from the superior colliculus and occipital striate cortex, sending projections to the primary and secondary visual cortices.

Further Reading: Moore and Psaaros. Definitive neurologic surgery board review, 2005, page 39.

Greenstein B, Greenstein A, Color Atlas of Neuroscience, 2000, thalamic nuclei section.

13.

C CA3

The hippocampus is made of 4 regions. CA1, also known as Sommer's sector, is extremely sensitive to hypoxia, while CA3 is located at the genu of the hippocampal formation and is relatively resistant to hypoxia.

Further Reading: Greenstein B, Greenstein A. Color Atlas of Neuroscience, 2000, the hippocampus.

14.

A Foramen spinosum

The primary artery feeding the pachymeninges is the middle meningial artery, and it enters the skull through the foramen spinosum.

Further Reading: Moore and Psaaros. Definitive Neurologic Surgery Board Review, 2005, page 54.

Greenstein B, Greenstein A. Color Atlas of Neuroscience, 2000, brain vascularization, arterial supply.

15.

B Superior

In the roof of the third ventricle, the body of the fornix resides superior to the paired internal cerebral veins.

Further Reading: Greenstein B, Greenstein A. Color Atlas of Neuroscience, 2000, venous drainage of the brain.

16.

B Fornix

Part of the Papez circuit, the hypothalamus receives input from the hippocampus through the fornix, which projects to the hypothalamic septal, dorsal and lateral preoptic regions through the precommissural fibers, and to the mammillary bodies through the postcommissural fibers. Information is then sent to the thalamus through the mammillothalamic tract.

Further Reading: Moore and Psaaros. Definitive Neurologic Surgery Board Review, 2005, pages 44, 45.

Greenstein B, Greenstein A. Color Atlas of Neuroscience, 2000, the hippocampus.

17.

D Insular cortex

The amygdala is part of the limbic system and receives input from all structures mentioned above. By far, the largest input to the amygdala is through the insular cortex.

Further Reading: Moore and Psaaros. Definitive Neurologic Surgery Board Review, 2005, page 48.

Greenstein B, Greenstein A. Color Atlas of Neuroscience, 2000, functions of the amygdaloid complex.

18.

A Medial geniculate body

Brodmann areas 41 and 42 correspond to Heschel's gyrus, or the primary auditory cortex located in the superior temporal gyrus. The primary input is the medial geniculate body. The lateral geniculate body and superior colliculus are involved in visual pathways, while the inferior colliculus provides projections to the medial geniculate body via the brachium of the inferior colliculus.

Further Reading: Moore and Psaaros. Definitive Neurologic Surgery Board Review, 2005, page 28.

Greenstein B, Greenstein A. Color Atlas of Neuroscience, 2000, the special senses: auditory cortical areas and descending auditory pathways.

19.

C Left superior quadrantanopsia

The seizure semiology presented in this case is classic for temporal lobe epilepsy, often caused by mesial temporal sclerosis. The symptoms from this patient localize to the right temporal lobe. This condition can be treated by selective amygdalohippocampectomy, or even complete temporal lobectomy. On the left side, resection of cortex should not exceed 4 to 5 cm to avoid harming language function presumed to be on the left side near the angular gyrus. On the right side, resection can often be safely carried 6 to 7 cm posterior given that language function is not presumed to be located on the right side. Care must be taken at the posterior-superior aspect of the resection in this region, as aggressive resection can involve the optic radiations (Meyer's loop), causing the classic "pie in the sky" visual field cut, a contralateral superior quadrant anopsia.

Further Reading: Greenstein B, Greenstein A. Color Atlas of Neuroscience, 2000, the visual fields and pathways.

20.

A Lateral

The patient has Parkinsonism, and you are performing bilateral STN deep brain stimulation. If ipsilateral eye deviation is noticed during test stimulation, your electrode is too medial and needs to be moved lateral. Efferent fibers ultimately forming the IIIrd nerve pass just medial to the STN and can be stimulated causing eye deviation if the electrode is too medial.

Further Reading: Greenstein B, Greenstein A. Color Atlas of Neuroscience, 2000, oculomotor nuclei and nerves.

21.

B Posteromedial

Descending corticospinal motor neuron tracts from the internal capsule travel anterolateral to STN. If contralateral facial pulling or muscle twitching is noted during test stimulation, the electrode is too far in the anterior or lateral position and should be moved posteromedially.

Further Reading: Greenstein B, Greenstein A. Color Atlas of Neuroscience, 2000, descending motor tracts and cranial nerve nuclei.

22.

A Lateral

The most commonly targeted nucleus for patients with dystonia is GPI. If the DBS electrode is too medial, stimulation current can spread to the internal capsule, which is medial to the GPI nucleus. The electrode should be moved laterally.

Further Reading: Greenstein B, Greenstein A. Color Atlas of Neuroscience, 2000, cerebral hemispheres: internal structures.

23.

B Superior

If a patient develops phosphenes in their visual field (flashing lights), it indicates that the electrode is too deep. Optic pathways run inferior to the GPI nuclei, and the electrode should be moved superiorly.

Further Reading: Greenstein B, Greenstein A. Color Atlas of Neuroscience, 2000, cerebral hemispheres: internal structures.

24.

C Medial

For essential tremor, DBS electrode placement into bilateral VIM thalamus has shown excellent results. The internal capsule is lateral to the thalamus, and if your patient develops muscle contractions, you should move the electrode medially.

Further Reading: Greenstein B, Greenstein A. Color Atlas of Neuroscience, 2000, origin of the pyramidal tract.

25.

A Anterior

VIM thalamus is just anterior to the VPL nucleus of the thalamus, the main sensory relay nucleus of the thalamus. If the electrode is placed correctly into VIM, patients can develop transient paresthesias during test stimulation, but these symptoms often resolve quite quickly. If the patient develops persistent paresthesias, current is likely spreading into VPL thalamus, and the electrode should be moved anteriorly.

Further Reading: Israel, Burchiel, Microelectrode Recording in Movement Disorder Surgery, 2004, target selection using microelectrode recording.

26.

D Anteroinferior

Utilizing the MCA M1 segment to reach the ICA terminus is one technique to expose an ICA terminus aneurysm. The main concern dissecting along the M1 segment of the MCA is preservation of the lateral lenticulostriate perforating arteries, which are located on the posterosuperior aspect of the M1 segment. The safe zone of dissection is on the anteroinferior surface of the vessel.

Further Reading: Spetzler, Kalani, Nakaji. Neurovascular Surgery, 2nd edition, 2015, surgical therapies for saccular aneurysms of the internal carotid artery.

27.

B Limen insulae

The limen insula is a structure that connects the temporal and orbital cortical regions. It often marks the MCA bifurcation, and laterally is continuous with the insular cortex. Medially it is bordered by the anterior perforated substance.

Further Reading: Starr, Barbaro, Larson, Neurosurgical Operative Atlas: Functional Neurosurgery, 2nd edition, 2009, surgical anatomy of the temporal lobe.

28.

A Cingulate gyrus

The cingulate gyrus is located immediately superior to the corpus callosum, and must be gently retracted to expose the corpus callosum for division. Care must be taken to avoid damaging the pericallosal arteries, which are also running immediately over the corpus callosum

Further Reading: Sekhar, Fessler, Atlas of Neurosurgical Techniques: Brain, Vol. 2, 2016, surgical approaches to lesions located in the lateral, third, and fourth ventricles.

29.

D Thalamostriate vein

The vein of Galen may have numerous supplying veins, but most often it receives the paired internal cerebral veins, the paired basal veins of Rosenthal and the precentral cerebellar vein. The thalamostriate vein of the lateral ventricle drains into the internal cerebral vein at the venous angle near the foramen of Monro, but this vein does not directly drain into the vein of Galen.

Further Reading: Spetzler, Kalani, Nakaji. Neurovascular Surgery, 2nd edition, 2015, microsurgical treatment of vein of Galen malformations.

30.

A Anterior

During an endoscopic third ventriculostomy, one of the easiest structures to identify are the paired mammillary bodies. Just anterior to the mammillary bodies is the safe zone for puncture. Care must be taken to not injure the basilar artery or posterior cerebellar arteries, which are just deep and slightly posterior to the puncture location

Further Reading: Torres-Corzo, Rangel-Castilla, Nakaji. Neuroendoscopic Surgery, 2016, lateral and third ventricle anatomy.

31.

B Lamina terminalis

In the anterior floor of the third ventricle, the lamina terminalis is located superior to the supraoptic recess. It is formed during closure of the anterior neuropore on embryological day 24. Division of the lamina terminalis allows access to the third ventricle for drainage of CSF and brain relaxation if required during anterior fossa aneurysm surgery.

Further Reading: Torres-Corzo, Rangel-Castilla, Nakaji. Neuroendoscopic, Surgery, 2016, lateral and third ventricle anatomy.

32.

C Lambdoid

The lambdoid suture connects the occipital and parietal bones while descending laterally across the posterior skull.

Further Reading: Greenberg. Handbook of Neurosurgery, 8th edition, 2016, gross anatomy, cranial and spine.

33.

D Coronal-sagittal

The bregma is a midline skull structure that is the location where the coronal and sagittal sutures conjoin. It is the location of the anterior fontanelle, which closes in most pediatric patients around 18 months of age.

Further Reading: Greenberg. Handbook of Neurosurgery, 8th edition, 2016, gross anatomy, cranial and spine.

34.

D Vestibular

The deep cerebellar nuclei are the dentate, emboliform, globose and fastigial, going from lateral to medial. A mnemonic to remember is "Don't Eat Greasy Foods." Since the deep cerebellar nuclei control all output from the cerebellum, damage to these structures can mimic a complete cerebellar resection and are considered by some to be "eloquent cortex."

Further Reading: Psarros. The Definitive Neurosurgical Board Review.

Alberstone, Benzel, Najm, Steinmetz. Anatomic Basis of Neurologic Diagnosis, 2009, cerebellum.

35.

A Brachium conjunctivum

The 4th ventricle has lateral walls formed superiorly by the superior cerebellar peduncle (brachium conjunctivis), and lateral walls formed inferiorly by the inferior cerebellar peduncle (restiform body). The middle cerebellar peduncle (brachium pontis) does not form a lateral wall of the 4th ventricle. The roof of the 4th ventricle is formed by both the superior and inferior medullary velum, and the floor is formed by the brainstem.

Further Reading: Psarros. The Definitive Neurosurgical Board Review.

Alberstone, Benzel, Najm, Steinmetz. Anatomic Basis of Neurologic Diagnosis, 2009, cerebellum.

36.

B Restiform body

The 4th ventricle has lateral walls formed superiorly by the superior cerebellar peduncle (brachium conjunctivis), and lateral walls formed inferiorly by the inferior cerebellar peduncle (restiform body). The middle cerebellar peduncle (brachium pontis) does not form a lateral wall of the 4th ventricle. The roof of the 4th ventricle is formed by both the superior and inferior medullary velum, and the floor is formed by the brainstem.

Further Reading: Psarros. The Definitive Neurosurgical Board Review.

Alberstone, Benzel, Najm, Steinmetz. Anatomic Basis of Neurologic Diagnosis, 2009, cerebellum.

37.

D Flocculonodular lobe

The cerebellum can be divided in to three functional segments, the vestibulocerebellum, the spinocerebellum and the cerebrocerebellum. The vestibulocerebellum is formed by the flocculonodular lobe and it receives projections from the vestibular nuclei, the superior colliculi and visual cortex. This system controls head and eye movements as well as postural and balance adjustments.

Further Reading: Psarros. The Definitive Neurosurgical Board Review, page 37.

Alberstone, Benzel, Najm, Steinmetz. Anatomic Basis of Neurologic Diagnosis, 2009, cerebellum.

38.

B Lateral hemisphere

The functional division of the cerebellum known as the cerebrocerebellum is comprised of the lateral hemispheres. It projects to the dentate nucleus of the deep cerebellar nuclei. Further connections include the VL nuclei of the thalamus and red nucleus, followed by motor cortex, and helps to provide feedback to motor cortex regarding accuracy of movement.

Further Reading: Psarros. The Definitive Neurosurgical Board Review, page 37.

Alberstone, Benzel, Najm, Steinmetz. Anatomic Basis of Neurologic Diagnosis, 2009, cerebellum.

39.

C Vermis

The functional division of the cerebellum known as the spinocerebellum is comprised mainly of the vermis. It projects to the fastigial nucleus of the deep cerebellar nuclei. It receives afferent connections from the spinocerebellar tract. Efferent connections from the fastigial nucleus project to the reticular formation and lateral vestibular nuclei, as well as the contralateral motor cortex via the VL thalamus.

Further Reading: Psarros. The Definitive Neurosurgical Board Review, page 37.

Alberstone, Benzel, Najm, Steinmetz. Anatomic Basis of Neurologic Diagnosis, 2009, cerebellum.

40.

B Abducens nucleus

The paramedian pontine reticular formation is also known as the lateral gaze center, and it is located near the abducens nucleus. It receives input from the superior colliculus to coordinate vertical eye movements, and from the frontal eye fields via the frontopontine fibers to coordinate lateral gaze. Contralateral eye movement in a conjugate fashion is mediated by crossing fibers from the medial longitudinal fasciculus.

Further Reading: Psarros. The Definitive Neurosurgical Board Review, page 33.

Alberstone, Benzel, Najm, Steinmetz. Anatomic Basis of Neurologic Diagnosis, 2009, brainstem.

41.

B Medial longitudinal fasciculus

In this scenario, the patient is not able to adduct the right eye when attempting to look left, while the left eye is able to abduct. This likely represents a lesion of the medial longitudinal fasciculus.

Further Reading: Psarros. The Definitive Neurosurgical Board Review, page 32.

Alberstone, Benzel, Najm, Steinmetz. Anatomic Basis of Neurologic Diagnosis, 2009, vestibular system.

42.

B Facial colliculus

The paired facial colliculi form noticeable structures on surface of the floor of the 4th ventricle. They are located above the bilateral stria medullari. Care should be taken to not violate the floor of the 4th ventricle.

Further Reading: Binder, Sonne, Fischbein. Cranial Nerves: Anatomy, Pathology, Imaging, 2010, facial nerve.

43.

B Lateral

There are several observable structures on the surface of the floor of the 4th ventricle. The paired facial colliculi are prominences that can be seen above the laterally projecting fibers of the stria medullari. Below the stria, the hypoglossal trigone is closest to midline, with the vagal trigone located lateral to the hypoglossal trigone.

Further Reading: Binder, Sonne, Fischbein. Cranial Nerves: Anatomy, Pathology, Imaging, 2010, vagus nerve.

44.

B Internal arcuate fibers

The nuclei gracilis and cuneatus receive sensory input from the dorsal columns of the spinal cord. In the medulla they decussate and form the medial lemniscus. The decussating fibers cross the midline as internal arcuate fibers.

Further Reading: Psarros. The Definitive Neurologic Surgery Board Review, page 30.

Citow, Macdonald, Refai. Comprehensive Neurosurgery Board Review, 2nd edition, 2010, anatomy.

45.

A Area prostrema

The circumventricular organs are regions of the brain located at the boundaries of the ventricular system and they are regions with an incomplete blood brain barrier. This allows these regions to sense peptide levels within the brain without requiring active transport mechanisms. There circumventricular organs include the median eminence, posterior pituitary, subcommissural organ, subforniceal organ, area prostrema, choroid plexus, vascular organ of the lamina terminalis and pineal gland. The only paired circumventricular organ is the area prostrema.

Further Reading: Psarros. The definitive Neurologic Surgery Board Review, page 30.

Yaşargil, Adamson, Cravens, Johnson, Reeves, Teddy, Valavanis, Wichmann, Wild, Young. Microneurosurgery IV A, 1994, neurophysiology.

46.

C Laterally

The cerebral peduncles contain descending corticospinal tracts organized in a somatotopic organization with the sacral fibers occupying the most lateral aspect of the corticospinal tracts, and fibers controlling the head/arms are the most medial.

Further Reading: Psarros. The Definitive Neurologic Surgery Board Review, page 34.

Alberstone, Benzel, Najm, Steinmetz. Anatomic Basis of Neurologic Diagnosis, 2009, brainstem.

47.

B Superior colliculi

The nucleus of the IIIrd nerve, the occulomotor nucleus, is located roughly at the same horizontal level as the superior colliculi.

Further Reading: Psarros. The Definitive Neurologic Surgery Board Review, page 34.

Alberstone, Benzel, Najm, Steinmetz. Anatomic Basis of Neurologic Diagnosis, 2009, brainstem.

48.

C Pretectal

The pretectal nucleus controls the direct and consensual pupillary light reflex

Further Reading: Psarros. The Definitive Neurologic Surgery Board Review, page 34.

Alberstone, Benzel, Najm, Steinmetz. Anatomic Basis of Neurologic Diagnosis, 2009, visual system.

49.

A Subcommissural organ

The subcommissural organ is made of ependymal cells that secrete somatostatin. It is the only circumventricular organ with an intact blood brain barrier.

Further Reading: Psarros. The Definitive Neurologic Surgery Board Review, page 34.

Yaşargil, Adamson, Cravens, Johnson, Reeves, Teddy, Valavanis, Wichmann, Wild, Young. Microneurosurgery IV A, 1994, neurophysiology.

50.

D Medial lemniscus

The medial lemniscus appears as a curved structure projecting laterally from the red nucleus on a horizontal section through the midbrain.

Further Reading: Psarros. The Definitive Neurologic Surgery Board Review, page 35.

Alberstone, Benzel, Najm, Steinmetz. Anatomic Basis of Neurologic Diagnosis, 2009, brainstem.

51.

C Superior cerebellar artery

The deep cerebellar nuclei are located very close to the superior cerebellar peduncle within the vicinity of the superior lateral wall of the 4th ventricle. The superior cerebellar artery provides blood supply to the superior surface of the cerebellum as well as to the superior cerebellar peduncle and the majority of the deep cerebellar nuclei.

Further Reading: Psarros. The Definitive Neurologic Surgery Board Review, page 38.

Spetzler, Kalani, Nakaji. Neurovascular Surgery, 2nd edition, 2015, cranial vascular anatomy of the posterior circulation.

52.

C Medial

At the level of the midbrain, the descending corticospinal tracts are located in the ventral region of the midbrain and are arranged in a somatotopic fashion. The tracts controlling the upper extremity are located medial to tracts controlling lower extremity function.

Further Reading: Alberstone, Benzel, Najm, Steinmetz. Anatomic Basis of Neurologic Diagnosis, 2009, brainstem.

53.

A Medial

At the level of the medulla, after the internal arcuate fibers have crossed and formed the medial lemniscus, the fibers conveying information from the upper extremity are located dorsal and the fibers from the lower extremity are located ventrally. As these fibers ascend to the level of the midbrain, the medial lemniscus becomes a curve structure extending laterally from the red nucleus. In this region, the fibers from the upper extremity are the most medial, while the lower extremity fibers are located laterally.

Further Reading: Alberstone, Benzel, Najm, Steinmetz. Anatomic Basis of Neurologic Diagnosis, 2009, brainstem.

54.

D Nasociliary nerve

The annulus of Zinn is a structure located in the superior orbital fissure, dividing it into sections. There are multiple structures that pass through the annulus of Zinn, including the oculomotor nerve, the nasociliary nerve, the abducens nerve and roots of the ciliary ganglion. The frontal nerve, trochlear nerve and lacrimal nerve all pass outside of the annulus of Zinn.

Further Reading: Citow, Macdonald, Refai. Comprehensive Neurosurgery Board Review, 2nd edition, 2010, anatomy.

55.

C Superior oblique palsy

The IVth nerve (trochelar nerve), runs at the edge of the tentorial incisura in the ambient cistern and is at risk during complete division of the tentorium.

Further Reading: Binder, Sonne, Fischbein. Cranial Nerves: Anatomy, Pathology, Imaging, 2010, trochlear nerve.

56.

B Nystagmus to the left

Cold calorics involve irrigating cold saline into the patient's ear and observing the movements of the eyes. The mnemonic COWS (cold-opposite, warm-same) is useful to remember, but it must be noted that this mnemonic refers to the nystagmus portion of the eye movements. In this patient, you irrigate the right ear with cold saline, and you would expect a slow drift of the eyes to the right followed by a fast-jerk nystagmus back to the left. The cold saline decreases the temperature of the tympanic membrane and hyperpolarizes the vestibular cells, tricking the system into thinking the head is moving to the left.

Further Reading: Alberstone, Benzel, Najm, Steinmetz. Anatomic Basis of Neurologic Diagnosis, 2009, vestibular system.

57.

A Base

The cochlea is a coiled organ that process auditory input. It is arranged tonotopically with high frequency sounds processed at the base, and low-frequency sounds processed at the apex.

Further Reading: Alberstone, Benzel, Najm, Steinmetz. Anatomic Basis of Neurologic Diagnosis, 2009, auditory system.

58.

A Tectorial membrane

As sound travels through the cochlea it causes movement of the basilar membrane, which in turn moves the organ of Corti at specific locations. This movement causes a shearing motion against the tectorial membrane, to which the ciliary processes of the hair cells are connected. This movement causes opening of these processes and depolarization of the hair cells

Further Reading: Alberstone, Benzel, Najm, Steinmetz. Anatomic Basis of Neurologic Diagnosis, 2009, auditory system.

59.

C Ventral cochlear nucleus–superior olive

The trapezoid body conveys information from the cochlear nucleus to the superior olive. Fibers then travel to the inferior colliculus and subsequently the medial geniculate body.

Further Reading: Alberstone, Benzel, Najm, Steinmetz. Anatomic Basis of Neurologic Diagnosis, 2009, auditory system.

60.

C Lateral lemniscus

The lateral lemniscus connects the dorsal cochlear nucleus to the inferior colliculus via the lateral lemniscus. It is involved in the response to sudden loud noises.

Further Reading: Alberstone, Benzel, Najm, Steinmetz. Anatomic Basis of Neurologic Diagnosis, 2009, auditory system.

61.

A Spinal trigeminal nucleus

The corneal blink reflex pathway involves sensory information from the cornea passing through the trigeminal nerve to the spinal trigeminal nucleus and tract. Further connections include the bilateral facial nuclei which mediate eye closure.

Further Reading: Rohkamm. Color Atlas of Neurology, 2007, normal and abnormal function of the nervous system.

62.

B Facial nerve

Fibers traveling from the facial nucleus travel around the abducens nucleus in the brainstem.

Further Reading: Binder, Sonne, Fischbein. Cranial Nerves: Anatomy, Pathology, Imaging, 2010, facial nerve.

63.

B Ventromedial

The ventromedial nucleus of the hypothalamus controls satiety. A way to remember this is "if the ventromedial nucleus is destroyed, you grow ventrally and medially."

Further Reading: Alberstone, Benzel, Najm, Steinmetz. Anatomic Basis of Neurologic Diagnosis, 2009, hypothalamus.

64.

D Supraoptic

The supraoptic nuclei of the hypothalamus are involved in fluid balance regulation.

Further Reading: Alberstone, Benzel, Najm, Steinmetz. Anatomic Basis of Neurologic Diagnosis, 2009, hypothalamus.

65.

A Central tegmental tract

Gustatory information from the tongue and oropharynx travels through the chorda tympani and VIIth nerve, as well as the IX/X nerves. 1st order neurons synapse in the nucleus of the solitary tract. Then, 2nd order neurons travel via the central tegmental tract to VPM thalamus and 3rd order neurons travel from VPM thalamus to the postcentral gyrus.

Further Reading: Greenstein B, Greenstein A. Color Atlas of Neuroscience, 2000, transverse section of medulla oblongata II.

66.

C Superior olivary nucleus

The auditory dampening reflex is mediated by the superior olivary nucleus and involves contraction of the stapedius (VIIth nerve) and tensor tympani (Vth nerve).

Further Reading: Psarros. Intensive neurosurgery board review.

Greenstein B, Greenstein A. Color Atlas of Neuroscience, 2000, localization of sound.

67.

B Ethmoid bone

The cribiform plate is a bony structure that is part of the ethmoid bone in the anterior cranial fossa. It supports the olfactory bulb and has numerous foramina through which the olfactory nerves pass to reach the nose.

Further Reading: Wanibuchi, Friedman, Fukushima. Photo Atlas of Skull Base Dissection, 2009, craniofacial anatomy.

68.

B Maxillary nerve

The maxillary nerve, or V2, does not pass through the superior orbital fissure.

Further Reading: Di Ieva, Lee, Cusimano. Handbook of Skull Base Surgery, 2016, clinical and neurologic findings in skull base pathology.

69.

B Pars vascularis of the jugular foramen

The vagus nerve exits the skull through the jugular foramen, which is divided into two regions by the jugular spine, the pars nervosa (carrying the glossopharyngeal nerve and inferior petrosal sinus) and the pars vascularis (carrying the jugular bulb, vagus nerve and spinal accessory nerve).

Further Reading: Binder, Sonne, Fischbein. Cranial Nerves: Anatomy, Pathology, Imaging, 2010, vagus nerve.

70.

C Foramen spinosum

The middle meningeal artery is the most common offending artery in cases of epidural hematoma. It enters the skull as a branch from the internal maxillary artery through the foramen spinosum.

Further Reading: Wanibuchi, Friedman, Fukushima. Photo Atlas of Skull Base Dissection, 2009, middle fossa rhomboid approach (anterior petrosectomy).

71.

D Ophthalmic artery

The anterior and posterior ethmoidal arteries give blood supply to the mucosal surfaces of the ethmoid bone, and they are both branches from the ophthalmic artery.

Further Reading: Spetzler, Kalani, Nakaji. Neurovascular Surgery, 2nd edition, 2015, microsurgical anatomy of the internal carotid and vertebral arteries.

72.

D Sphenopalatine artery

The sphenopalatine artery gives blood supply to the middle turbinate, which can be removed by an access surgeon to allow expanded access for endoscopic approaches to the sella and anterior skull base.

Further Reading: Stamm. Transnasal Endoscopic Skull Base and Brain Surgery, 2011, anatomy of the nasal cavity and paranasal sinuses.

73.

A Optic strut

The optic strut joins the lesser wing of the sphenoid to the body of the sphenoid bone. It forms the inferior and lateral wall of the optic canal. It separates the optic canal from the superior orbital fissure. From an endonasal approach, it is located inferior to the optic protuberence, superiomedial to the carotid protuberence, and medial to the lateral opticocarotid recess.

Further Reading: Laws, Sheehan. Sellar and Parasellar Tumors, 2012, anatomy of the sellar and parasellar region.

74.

B Planum sphenoidale

Just anterosuperior to the sella turcica is the planum sphenoidale. This can be a site of meningioma growth, and tumors in this region can be accessed via an expanded endonasal approach.

Further Reading: Di Ieva, Lee, Cusimano. Handbook of Skull Base Surgery, 2016, anatomy of the skull base and related structures: elements of surgical anatomy.

75.

B Greater superficial petrosal nerve

The vidian nerve is continuous with the greater superficial petrosal nerve and passes through the vidian canal lateral to the ethmoid air cells. The vidian nerve carries sensory fibers from the facial nerve supplying the soft palate. It is an important landmark in endoscopic endonasal surgery as it leads directly to the carotid artery.

Further Reading: Di Ieva, Lee, Cusimano. Handbook of Skull Base Surgery, 2016, anatomy of the skull base and related structures: elements of surgical anatomy.

76.

B Foramen rotundum

The foramen rotundum is just lateral to the vidian canal and contains the maxillary nerve. Both the vidian canal and foramen rotundum are openings in the greater wing of the sphenoid bone. In this location they connect the middle cranial fossa to the pterygopalatine fossa.

Further Reading: Di Ieva, Lee, Cusimano. Handbook of Skull Base Surgery, 2016, anatomy of the skull base and related structures: elements of surgical anatomy.

77.

D Abducens nerve

The cavernous sinus contains several nerves, including CN III, IV, V1, and VI. All nerves run in the lateral wall of the cavernous sinus except for the abducens nerve, which runs with the carotid artery through the cavernous sinus.

Further Reading: Di Ieva, Lee, Cusimano. Handbook of Skull Base Surgery, 2016, anatomy of the skull base and related structures: elements of surgical anatomy.

78.

A Glasscock's triangle

The posterolateral triangle of the skull base is bordered by V3 (mandibular nerve), the greater superficial petrosal nerve, and a line drawn between the foramen spinosum and the arcuate eminence. This triangle can be important during skull base neurosurgery given that it allows for the exposure of the horizontal segment of the petrous internal carotid artery by drilling out bone inferior to the border of V3.

Further Reading: Di Ieva, Lee, Cusimano. Handbook of Skull Base Surgery, 2016, anatomy of the skull base and related structures: elements of surgical anatomy.

79.

B Kawase's traingle

The posteromedial triangle of the skull base is bordered by V3 (mandibular nerve), the greater superficial petrosal nerve (inferiorly), and the superior petrosal sinus. This triangle can be important during skull base neurosurgery given that drilling in this region allows for an anterior petrosectomy, connecting the middle and posterior cranial fossae. It contains the petrous corner of the ICA and in its lateral aspect contains the cochlea.

Further Reading: Di Ieva, Lee, Cusimano. Handbook of Skull Base Surgery, 2016, anatomy of the skull base and related structures: elements of surgical anatomy.

80.

C Infratrochlear triangle

The infratrochlear triangle (Parkinson's triangle) of the skull base is bordered by the trochlear nerve (superior), V1, and the tentorial edge. This triangle can be important during skull base neurosurgery as it contains the horizontal segment of the cavernous carotid, the abducens nerve and the meningohypophyseal trunk. It has been described as the original access location to the cavernous sinus.

Further Reading: Di Ieva, Lee, Cusimano. Handbook of Skull Base Surgery, 2016, anatomy of the skull base and related structures: elements of surgical anatomy.

81.

B Superior vestibular nerve–inferior vestibular nerve

Bill's bar is a vertically oriented bone within the IAC that separates the Facial nerve (anterosuperior) from the superior vestibular nerve (posterosuperior). The cochlear nerve is located anteroinferior, and the inferior vestibular nerve is located posteroinferior.

Further Reading: Di Ieva, Lee, Cusimano. Handbook of Skull Base Surgery, 2016, anatomy of the skull base and related structures: elements of surgical anatomy.

82.

C Anterior inferior cerebellar artery

The posterior fossa can be thought of as three distinct neurovascular regions. The superior region contains CN III, IV, and V, and is associated with the superior cerebellar artery. The middle neurovascular region consists of CN VI, VII, and VIII as well as the anterior inferior cerebellar artery. The inferior neurovascular region contains CN IX, X, XI, and XII, and is associated with the posterior inferior cerebellar artery.

Further Reading: Di Ieva, Lee, Cusimano. Handbook of Skull Base Surgery, 2016, anatomy of the skull base and related structures: elements of surgical anatomy.

83.

D Asterion

The asterion is located where the squamous and parietomastoid sutures join. It is a rough landmark for the transverse sigmoid sinus, and can be an important marker for burr hole location in retrosigmoid craniectomies.

Further Reading: Di Ieva, Lee, Cusimano. Handbook of Skull Base Surgery, 2016, anatomy of the skull base and related structures: elements of surgical anatomy.

84.

B Trochlear

The trochlear nerve is the only cranial nerve to exit from the dorsal aspect of the brainstem.

Further Reading: Binder, Sonne, Fischbein. Cranial Nerves: Anatomy, Pathology, Imaging, 2010, trochlear nerve.

85.

B Mesoderm

The meninges of the skull base arise from the mesoderm of the embryo. This differs from telencephalic meninges which arise from neural crest cells.

Further Reading: Di Ieva, Lee, Cusimano. Handbook of Skull Base Surgery, 2016, skull base embryology.

86.

D Labyrinthine artery

The labyrinthine artery is most commonly a branch from the anterior inferior cerebellar artery, and it follows the vestibulocochlear nerve into the IAC.

Further Reading: Di Ieva, Lee, Cusimano. Handbook of Skull Base Surgery, 2016, anatomy of the skull base and related structures: elements of surgical anatomy.

87.

B Ophthalmic artery

The ophthalmic artery originates from the internal carotid just distal to the distal dural ring, making it the first intradural branch of the internal carotid artery.

Further Reading: Di Ieva, Lee, Cusimano. Handbook of Skull Base Surgery, 2016, anatomy of the skull base and related structures: elements of surgical anatomy.

88.

C Olfactory nerve

Special visceral afferent fibers conveying sense of smell travel through the olfactory nerve directly to the primary olfactory areas via the medial and lateral olfactory striae.

Further Reading: Psarros. The Definitive Neurosurgical Board Review.

Binder, Sonne, Fischbein. Cranial Nerves: Anatomy, Pathology, Imaging, 2010, olfactory nerve.

89.

A Ganglion cells

Within the retina, the bioplar cells are the primary sensory neurons. The ganglion cells receive input from bipolar cells, and the axons of the ganglion cells make up the optic nerve.

Further Reading: Psarros. The Definitive Neurosurgical Board Review.

Binder, Sonne, Fischbein. Cranial Nerves: Anatomy, Pathology, Imaging, 2010, optic nerve.

90.

A Inferior oblique

The oculomotor nerve begins within the oculomotor nucleus at the level of the superior colliculus. It travels between the PCA and SCA and enters the orbit through the superior orbital fissure. Notably, it does travel within the annulus of Zinn. It separates into a superior division and inferior division, with the superior division innervating the levator palpebrae and superior rectus, while the inferior division innervates the medial/inferior rectus and the inferior oblique.

Further Reading: Psarros. The Definitive Neurosurgical Board Review.

Binder, Sonne, Fischbein. Cranial Nerves: Anatomy, Pathology, Imaging, 2010, oculomotor nerve.

91.

C Left trochlear nucleus

The trochlear nerve innervates the superior oblique muscle, and patients tend to tilt their head to the contralateral side of nerve injury to compensate. Also, the trochlear nerve is the only nerve to deccusate outside of the CNS, and the only cranial nerve to exit dorsally from the brainstem. This patient tilts her head to the left, meaning she would have sustained damage to either the right trochlear nerve (postdecussation), or the left trochlear nucleus (predecussation)

Further Reading: Psarros. The Definitive Neurosurgical Board Review.

Binder, Sonne, Fischbein. Cranial Nerves: Anatomy, Pathology, Imaging, 2010, trochlear nerve.

92.

A Trigeminal nerve

The trigeminal nerve has a portio major (sensory afferents from the face) and a portio minor (motor efferents) that travels with V3. The motor branch of the trigeminal nerve innervates the muscles of mastication, including the tensor veli palatini, masseter, pterygoids, temporalis and anterior belly of the digastric. It also innervates the tensor tympani, which dampens sudden loud noises in the efferent arm of the auditory reflex.

Further Reading: Psarros. The Definitive Neurosurgical Board Review.

Binder, Sonne, Fischbein. Cranial Nerves: Anatomy, Pathology, Imaging, 2010, trigeminal nerve.

93.

D Right abducens nucleus

The abducens nerve innervates the lateral rectus muscle and mediates lateral gaze of the ipsilateral eye. It is important to note that the abducens nucleus plays an important role in conjuage movement of the eyes. Signals initially reach the ipsilateral PPRF, which synapses on the ipsilateral abducens nucleus to mediate lateral gaze. The abducens nucleus also sends fibers to the contralateral oculomotor nucleus via the MLF to mediate conjugate medial deviation of the contralateral eye. Since this patient cannot cross midline with the left eye, the lesion must be within the abducens nucleus.

Further Reading: Psarros. The Definitive Neurosurgical Board Review.

Binder, Sonne, Fischbein. Cranial Nerves: Anatomy, Pathology, Imaging, 2010, abducens nerve.

94.

A Efferent arm of the corneal reflex

The facial nerve contains a large motor branch as well as a smaller branch known as the nervus intermedius. The motor branch controls muscles of facial expression and forehead. The nervus intermedius carries parasympathetic fibers to the lacrimal gland through the GSPN and pterygopalatine ganglion, parasympathetic fibers to the submandibular gland via the submandibular ganglion, and taste afferents via the chorda tympani. The efferent arm of the corneal reflex is mediated by muscles of facial expression and is carried in the motor branch of the facial nerve.

Further Reading: Psarros. The Definitive Neurosurgical Board Review.

Binder, Sonne, Fischbein. Cranial Nerves: Anatomy, Pathology, Imaging, 2010, facial nerve.

95.

B Spiral–cochlear

Hair cells from the organ of Corti within the cochlea synapse on the spiral ganglion, which in turn connects to the cochlear nucleus in the brainstem via the cochlear nerve. Scarpa's ganglion receives input from the receptors in the labyrinth of the saccule, utricle and semicircular canals. In turn, these fibers are transmitted to the vestibular nuclei of the brainstem via the vestibular nerve. Some fibers from Scarpa's ganglion travel to the flocculonodular lobe of the cerebellum as mossy fibers, where they mediate balance.

Further Reading: Psarros. The Definitive Neurosurgical Board Review.

Binder, Sonne, Fischbein. Cranial Nerves: Anatomy, Pathology, Imaging, 2010, vestibulocochlear nerve.

96.

A Lesser superficial petrosal nerve

The glossopharyngeal nerve innervates the parotid gland via branches that form the lesser superficial petrosal nerve. The lesser superficial petrosal nerve contains preganglionic parasympathetic nerves from the inferior salivatory nucleus of the brainstem that synapse in the otic ganglion. In turn, postganglionic parasympathetic nerves leave the otic ganglion and travel to the parotid gland via the auriculotemporal nerve (traveling with V3).

Further Reading: Psarros. The Definitive Neurosurgical Board Review.

Binder, Sonne, Fischbein. Cranial Nerves: Anatomy, Pathology, Imaging, 2010, glossopharyngeal nerve.

97.

D Cricothyroid

The recurrent laryngeal nerve is a branch from the vagus nerve that passes anterior to the subclavian artery on the right, and adjacent to the aorta on the left. Its recurrent route traverses in the tracheoesophageal groove. It innervates all intrinsic muscles of the larynx with the exception of the cricothyroid muscle.

Further Reading: Psarros. The Definitive Neurosurgical Board Review.

Binder, Sonne, Fischbein. Cranial Nerves: Anatomy, Pathology, Imaging, 2010, vagus nerve.

98.

C Posterior

The spinal accessory nerve has both a cranial and spinal point of origination. It innervates the sternocleidomastoid and trapezius muscles. The spinal portion passes posterior to the dentate ligament.

Further Reading: Psarros. The Definitive Neurosurgical Board Review.

Binder, Sonne, Fischbein. Cranial Nerves: Anatomy, Pathology, Imaging, 2010, spinal accessory nerve.

99.

A Palatoglossus

The hypoglossal nerve exits the brainstem between the inferior olive and the pyramids. It exits the skull via the hypoglossal canal and innervates all intrinsic and extrinsic muscles of the tongue except for the palatoglossus, which is innervated by the vagus nerve.

Further Reading: Psarros. The Definitive Neurosurgical Board Review.

Binder, Sonne, Fischbein. Cranial Nerves: Anatomy, Pathology, Imaging, 2010, hypoglossal nerve.

100.

D Rostral

The motor root of the trigeminal nerve most often arises rostral to the main sensory root of the trigeminal nerve.

Further Reading: Binder, Sonne, Fischbein. Cranial Nerves: Anatomy, Pathology, Imaging, 2010, trigeminal nerve.

11 Neurobiology

1.

B Anticholinergic

Oxybutynin is an anticholinergic drug that works on M1-3 muscarinic receptors in the bladder wall, inhibiting the activity of acetylcholine at this receptor. This leads to bladder relaxation which can help limit bladder spasticity and frequent urination.

Further Reading: Jallo, Vaccaro. Neurotrauma and Critical Care of the Spine, 2009, page 178.

Citow, Macdonald, Refai. Comprehensive Neurosurgery Board Review, 2nd edition, 2010.

2.

B Potassium

Astrocytes serve multiple functions in the brain, but they actively sequester potassium from the extracellular space in order to keep extracellular potassium levels low, thus maintaining the gradient of potassium required for membrane depolarization.

Further Reading: Jallo, Loftus. Neurotrauma and Critical Care of the Brain, 2009, page 34.

3.

C NMDA

The NMDA receptor utilizes glutamate as a ligand and after glutamate binds to the receptor, ion channels permeable to Na, K, and Ca open. It has been found to be associated with gene expression, synaptic plasticity, and other signaling systems. It is associated with pain, and ketamine is an NMDA receptor antagonist that can treat pain.

Further Reading: Burchiel. Surgical Management of Pain, 2nd edition, 2015, page 296.

Greenstein B, Greenstein A. Color Atlas of Neuroscience, 2000, page 108.

4.

E Supraoptic

The supraoptic nucleus of the hypothalamus is one of the anterior nuclei and is associated with ADH secretion from the posterior pituitary.

Further Reading: Greenstein B, Greenstein A. Color Atlas of Neuroscience, 2000, page 308.

5.

B Paraventricular

The supraoptic and paraventricular nuclei of the anterior hypothalamus are associated with secretion of ADH from the posterior pituitary. Of these two, the paraventricular nucleus also has diffuse connections to the spinal cord and brainstem.

Further Reading: Greenstein B, Greenstein A. Color Atlas of Neuroscience, 2000, page 308.

Greenstein B, Greenstein A. Color Atlas of Neuroscience, 2000, page 294.

6.

D Stress shielding

Wolf's law states that bone will form along lines of stress, and alternatively, when normal stress loads are removed, bone will become osteopenic. This is important in fusion surgery as the goal is for bone to heal across the fusion segment. If fixed angle screws are used both above and below the fusion segment, the bone may not be allowed to settle and put stress on the graft (which can lead to higher rates of fusion). If there is no stress on the graft, it is said to be "stress shielded" and the likelihood of fusion decreases.

Further Reading: Greenberg. The Handbook of Neurosurgery, 8th Edition, 2016, page 1091.

7.

A cGMP deactivation, hyperpolarization

Activation of rhodopsin is the final pathway in phototransduction. It deactivates cGMP via cGMP phosphodiesterase which has the effect of decreasing sodium ion movement across the cell membrane (occurs through cGMP associated Na channels). Ultimately this leads to hyperpolarization of the photoreceptor, and signal transduction.

Further Reading: Citow, Macdonald, Refai. Comprehensive Neurosurgery Board Review, 2nd edition, 2010, page 131.

Greenstein B, Greenstein A. Color Atlas of Neuroscience, 2000, page 276.

8.

E Layer VI

There are six cortical layers and cortical layer VI is associated projection fibers back to the thalamus. Layer IV receives input from the thalamus and is heavily myelinated in the occipital cortex (known as the stria of Gennari, also giving the name striate cortex). Layer V contains the large pyramidal Betz cells that project to the spinal cord.

Further Reading: Citow, Macdonald, Refai. Comprehensive Neurosurgery Board Review, 2nd edition, 2010, pages 32, 123.

9.

D Internal pyramidal

Betz cells of the cerebral cortex are large pyramidal neurons that project to the spinal cord. They are found in layer V, or the internal pyramidal layer of the cortex.

Further Reading: Citow, Macdonald, Refai. Comprehensive Neurosurgery Board Review, 2nd edition, 2010, pages 32, 123.

10.

B Potassium

TEA is a toxic compound that can lead to ganglionic competitive inhibition of acetylcholine. It also is known to block voltage gated potassium channels in nerve tissue and skeletal muscle.

Further Reading: Citow, Macdonald, Refai. Comprehensive Neurosurgery Board Review, 2nd edition, 2010, page 114.

11.

A Increased transmembrane resistance, decreased capacitance

Myelination of nerves helps to increase conduction velocity of the action potential. It increases the AP velocity by increasing transmembrane resistance and decreasing membrane capacitance.

Further Reading: Citow, Macdonald, Refai. Comprehensive Neurosurgery Board Review, 2nd edition, 2010, page 113.

12.

C Primary GBM

PTEN mutations are often seen in primary glioblastoma rather than low grade gliomas or secondary glioblastoma. For this reason it is helpful when determining if the GBM is primary or is representative of malignant transformation.

Further Reading: Gasco, Nader. The Essential Neurosurgery Companion, 2013, page 413.

13.

A Granular layer

The mossy fibers of the cerebellum synapse in the granular layer, and further projections arise from intrinsic cerebellar cortical cells. Only climbing fibers have direct synapses on Purkinje cells.

Further Reading: Alberstone, Benzel, Najm, Steinmetz. Anatomic Basis of Neurologic Diagnosis, 2009, page 283.

14.

B CA1–CA3

The intrinsic circuitry of the hippocampus is heavily tested. Mossy fibers connect the dentate gyrus to CA3, and the Schaffer collateral pathway interconnects the CA3 and CA1 regions.

Further Reading: Alberstone, Benzel, Najm, Steinmetz. Anatomic Basis of Neurologic Diagnosis, 2009, page 342.

15.

C Entorhinal cortex–dentate gyrus

The perforant pathway of the hippocampus is the initial limb of the intrinsic hippocampal circuitry. It initiates in the entorhinal cortex and perforates across the subiculum to enter the dentate gyrus.

Further Reading: Alberstone, Benzel, Najm, Steinmetz. Anatomic Basis of Neurologic Diagnosis, 2009, page 342.

16.

C Dopamine

The substantia nigra has two nuclei, pars reticulata and pars compacta. The pars compacta projects dopaminergic neurons to the striatum as part of the intrinsic basal ganglia circuitry.

Further Reading: Alberstone, Benzel, Najm, Steinmetz. Anatomic Basis of Neurologic Diagnosis, 2009, page 332.

17.

A Glutamate

The initial projections into the basal ganglia circuitry include motor cortex projections to the striatum. These projections are glutamatergic for both the direct and indirect pathways of the basal ganglia.

Further Reading: Alberstone, Benzel, Najm, Steinmetz. Anatomic Basis of Neurologic Diagnosis, 2009, page 332.

18.

B 3

The hippocampus has three layers which is considered archicortex, histologically older cortex than the cerebral cortex. The three layers are the molecular layer, the pyramidal layer, and the polymorphic layer.

Further Reading: Alberstone, Benzel, Najm, Steinmetz. Anatomic Basis of Neurologic Diagnosis, 2009, page 340.

19.

B Posterior nucleus

This patient is experiencing poikilothermia, or variance of body temperature with surrounding temperature. This is due to bilateral destruction of the posterior thalamic nucleus.

Further Reading: Yaşargil, Adamson, Cravens, Johnson, Reeves, Teddy, Valavanis, Wichmann, Wild, Young. Microneurosurgery IV A, 1994, page 268.

20.

C Hyperphagia

The ventromedial nucleus is involved in satiety and when bilaterally damaged, hyperphagia and obesity can occur. This is a known complication of complex craniopharyngioma resection in children and is a feared complication as it is very difficult to control in the postoperative setting.

Further Reading: Albright, Pollack, Adelson. Principles and Practice of Pediatric Neurosurgery, 3rd edition, 2015, page 490.

21.

A Anterior nucleus

The anterior hypothalamus is involved in cooling of the body and parasympathetic functions. The posterior nucleus is involved in sympathetic functions and heating.

Further Reading: Alberstone, Benzel, Najm, Steinmetz. Anatomic Basis of Neurologic Diagnosis, 2009, page 324.

22.

E D2

The medication you are using is haloperidol, a butyrophenone. It antagonizes both D1 and D2 receptors, but the D2 receptors are located in the frontal cortex, the limbic system, and the hippocampus. The D1 receptors are located in the striatum and are responsible for Parkinson-like effects of haloperidol.

Further Reading: Citow, Macdonald, Refai. Comprehensive Neurosurgery Board Review, 2nd edition, 2010, page 294.

23.

D Hypothalamus–intermediolateral cell column

Sympathetic innervation of the eye begins in the hypothalamus where first-order neurons project to the intermediolateral cell column. The second-order neuron connects the IML cell column to the superior cervical ganglion, and the third-order neuron connects the superior cervical ganglion to the radial musculature via long ciliary nerves.

Further Reading: Citow, Macdonald, Refai. Comprehensive Neurosurgery Board Review, 2nd edition, 2010, page 130.

24.

C Uncouples oxidative phosphorylation

Cyanide is a toxic compound that abolishes the proton gradient utilized during oxidative phosphorylation in the mitochondria. It leads to severe lactic acidosis and is highly toxic and ingestion is often fatal.

Further Reading: Meyers. Differential Diagnosis in Neuroimaging: Brain and Meninges, 2017, page 240.

Citow, Macdonald, Refai. Comprehensive Neurosurgery Board Review, 2nd edition, 2010, page 164.

25.

B Thoracic and abdominal viscera

The vagus nerve has multiple nuclei with different functions. The dorsal motor nucleus of the vagus nerve supplies visceral motor innervation of the thoracic and abdominal viscera, having parasympathetic functions on the gut.

Further Reading: Alberstone, Benzel, Najm, Steinmetz. Anatomic Basis of Neurologic Diagnosis, 2009, page 260.

26.

B G-protein

cAMP is a second messenger system within the G-protein receptor pathway. G proteins have three major subunits—alpha, beta, and gamma. The alpha subunit is associated with the interior plasma membrane and usually is the aspect that interacts with the effector enzymes. For G-protein receptors, G proteins are activated after GDP is exchanged for GTP. The G-proteins then stimulate adenylyl cyclase to synthesize cAMP which has downstream effects after it interacts with PKA (cAMP-dependent protein kinase), which in turn phosphorylates serine and threonine residues.

Further Reading: Psarros. The Definitive Neurosurgical Board Review, page 5.

Greenstein B, Greenstein A. Color Atlas of Neuroscience, 2000.

27.

B G_s

This patient has cholera, and cholera toxin selectively activates G_s, part of the G-protein signaling pathway.

Further Reading: Psarros. The Definitive Neurosurgical Board Review, page 5.

Greenstein B, Greenstein A. Color Atlas of Neuroscience, 2000.

28.

D IP_3

Inositol triphosphate (IP_3), is a messenger generated by DAG (along with phospholipase C), and is liberated from the plasma membrane through G-protein coupled messenger systems. IP_3 binds receptors in the mitochondria and ER causing Ca^{2+} to be released within the cytosol of the neuron.

Further Reading: Greenstein B, Greenstein A. Color Atlas of Neuroscience, 2000.

Psarros. The Definitive Neurosurgical Board Review, page 5.

29.

C NMDA

Nitric oxide liberation is a downstream effect of activation of the NMDA receptor signaling mechanism. NO is lipid soluble and in turn stimulates the production of cyclic-GMP.

Further Reading: Psarros. The Definitive Neurosurgical Board Review, page 5.

Greenstein B, Greenstein A. Color Atlas of Neuroscience, 2000.

30.

A Epidermal growth factor

Tyrosine kinase receptors bind ligands including epidermal growth factor, nerve growth factor, etc. Ultimately, binding of the ligands to this receptor subtype results in phosphorylation of serine and threonine residues. EGF receptor is often seen on high grade glial neoplasms, specifically astrocytic subtypes.

Further Reading: Psarros. The Definitive Neurosurgical Board Review, page 5.

Greenstein B, Greenstein A. Color Atlas of Neuroscience, 2000.

31.

A Alpha

The ACh receptor system is comprised of four major subunit types, with five total subunits—two alpha, one beta, one gamma, and one delta. Each alpha subunit binds one molecule of ACh, therefore requiring two molecules to activate the receptor.

Further Reading: Psarros. The Definitive Neurosurgical Board Review, page 6.

Greenstein B, Greenstein A. Color Atlas of Neuroscience, 2000.

32.

B Sodium influx into the cytosol

Alpha-bungarotoxin inhibits the alpha subunit of ACh receptors and in turn inhibits the influx of sodium into the cytosol.

Further Reading: Psarros. The Definitive Neurosurgical Board Review, page 6.

Greenstein B, Greenstein A. Color Atlas of Neuroscience, 2000.

33.

C Succinylcholine

Succinylcholine is a depolarizing neuromuscular blocking agent often used for intubation during induction of anesthesia. All other listed options are nondepolarizing agents.

Further Reading: Psarros. The Definitive Neurosurgical Board Review, page 6.

Greenstein B, Greenstein A. Color Atlas of Neuroscience, 2000.

34.

C Renshaw cells of the spinal cord

Muscarinic receptors are G-protein coupled receptors from the metabotropic family. They are inhibited by atropine and scopolamine, and activated by bethanechol and pilocarpine. They are located throughout the CNS, including the cortex, striatum, cerebellum, autonomic nuclei, and Renshaw cells of the spinal cord.

Further Reading: Psarros. The Definitive Neurosurgical Board Review, Page 6.

Greenstein B, Greenstein A. Color Atlas of Neuroscience, 2000.

35.

D $GABA_B$

The patient is suffering from baclofen withdrawal. Baclofen is a GABA agonist that works on the $GABA_B$ channel. Picrotoxin inhibits the $GABA_A$ receptor.

Further Reading: Psarros. The Definitive Neurosurgical Board Review, page 6.

Greenstein B, Greenstein A. Color Atlas of Neuroscience, 2000.

36.

C Neuregulin

There are a number of proteins that have effects on ACh receptor clustering in the NMJ. Neuregulin is responsible for increasing transcription of ACh receptors from within the muscle fiber, leading to increased concentration of these receptors in the NMJ.

Further Reading: Psarros. The Definitive Neurosurgical Board Review, page 10.

Greenstein B, Greenstein A. Color Atlas of Neuroscience, 2000.

37.

A Sarcoplasmic reticulum

After an action potential is generated at the NMJ, it propagates throughout the muscle cell and leads to release of Ca^{2+} from the sarcoplasmic reticulum.

Further Reading: Psarros. The Definitive Neurosurgical Board Review, page 11.

Greenstein B, Greenstein A. Color Atlas of Neuroscience, 2000.

38.

C Z disk

Each sarcomere is connected to another sarcomere at the Z disk. Unfortunately, elements of the sarcomere are often tested on the neurosurgical written boards.

Further Reading: Psarros. The Definitive Neurosurgical Board Review, page 11.

Greenstein B, Greenstein A. Color Atlas of Neuroscience, 2000.

39.

B H zone

During muscle contraction, Ca^{2+} facilitates crossbridges between actin/myosin fibrils. This leads to shortening of the H zone and the I band, while the A band remains the same size (this is because the actin fibrils move across the myosin fibrils and not the other way around).

Further Reading: Psarros. The Definitive Neurosurgical Board Review, page 11.

Greenstein B, Greenstein A. Color Atlas of Neuroscience, 2000.

40.

C Troponin C

Troponin C binds four molecules of Ca^{2+} within the muscle cell. This causes the troponin/tropomyosin complex to release from the actin fibril. In turn, this allows myosin heads to freely bind actin, forming the crossbridges. Next, myosin, which has

ATPase capability, rotates, pulling the actin fibril along its length, leading to muscle contraction. After this is complete, ATP binds myosin which recocks the myosin head, ready to grab the next actin binding site along the fibril.

Further Reading: Psarros. The Definitive Neurosurgical Board Review, page 11.

Greenstein B, Greenstein A. Color Atlas of Neuroscience, 2000.

41.

B Nonfunctioning pituitary adenoma

Imaging demonstrates a pituitary mass, and the lab work is suggestive of a nonfunctioning adenoma. Normal values for 8 AM cortisol are 6 to 14, the IGF-1 levels are within the normal range for a 40 year old (87 to 267), and the prolactin, while elevated (normal 3 to 30), is indicative of stalk effect rather than prolactinoma (> 150, but often much higher).

Further Reading: Greenberg. The Handbook of Neurosurgery, 8th edition, pages 733–736.

42.

D Neurohypophysis

This patient has central diabetes insipidus, caused by a lack of secretion of ADH from the posterior pituitary, or neurohypophysis. The diagnosis is made in the setting of consistent, high-volume urine output, dilute urine (specific gravity < 1.005), and increasing sodium levels. Patients can get profoundly dehydrated and may need administration of DDAVP.

Further Reading: Greenstein B, Greenstein A. Color Atlas of Neuroscience, 2000.

43.

D Hydrocortisone

This patient has Cushing's disease, most likely caused by an ACTH-secreting pituitary adenoma. If you are able to get a complete resection, it is important to give hydrocortisone as the patient can suffer an acute Addisonian crisis. Since the pituitary mass has inhibited endogenous production of ACTH, after complete resection, the source of ACTH will be eliminated and the endogenous steroid producing mechanisms have not yet ramped up. The patient will start feeling very nauseated and unwell, and blood pressure will be low. In such a case, 50 mg of IV hydrocortisone should be considered.

Further Reading: Greenstein B, Greenstein A. Color Atlas of Neuroscience, 2000.

44.

C Growth hormone

This patient has a growth-hormone secreting adenoma and may have features consistent with acromegaly. You should not order IGF-1 in the immediate postoperative period because it is similar to HgbA1c in that it represents levels of growth hormone over an extended period of time. You should order growth hormone to determine success of the surgery, as the levels of GH should respond much more quickly.

Further Reading: Greenberg. The Handbook of Neurosurgery, 8th edition, pages 733–736.

45.

B 50% reduction in cortisol levels after high dose DMZ suppression test

Patients with Cushing's disease will have a random ACTH > 5 ng/L, they will have a 50% or more reduction in cortisol levels after high dose DMZ test, often will have a positive IPS sampling (at least in the textbooks), and will have a positive metyrapone test (rise in 17-OHCS in urine 70% above baseline, or increase in serum 11-deoxycortisol 400-fold above normal).

Further Reading: Greenberg. The Handbook of Neurosurgery, 8th edition, page 735.

46.

B Dynein

Retrograde axonal transport is considered fast transport, occurring at roughly 400 mm/day. It utilizes ATP and the protein dynein.

Further Reading: Psarros. The Definitive Neurosurgical Board Review, page 3.

Greenstein B, Greenstein A. Color Atlas of Neuroscience, 2000.

Citow, Macdonald, Refai. Comprehensive Neurosurgery Board Review, 2nd edition, 2010, physiology section.

47.

D Kinesin

There are several types of slow anterograde axonal transport that utilize both dynamin and actin/myosin complexes. Fast anterograde transport utilizes kinesin and ATP, and can cover 400 mm/day.

Further Reading: Psarros. The Definitive Neurosurgical Board Review, page 2.

Greenstein B, Greenstein A. Color Atlas of Neuroscience, 2000.

Citow, Macdonald, Refai. Comprehensive Neurosurgery Board Review, 2nd edition, 2010, physiology section.

48.

C Vinblastine

Vinblastine is a chemotherapeutic agent that has the effect of limiting microtubule formation and function. This has the effect of inhibiting fast anterograde axonal transport as the protein kinesin utilizes microtubules and ATP during fast anterograde axonal transport.

Further Reading: Psarros. The Definitive Neurosurgical Board Review, page 2.

Greenstein B, Greenstein A. Color Atlas of Neuroscience, 2000.

Citow, Macdonald, Refai. Comprehensive Neurosurgery Board Review, 2nd edition, 2010, physiology section.

49.

B Norepinephrine

Norepinephrine is synthesized from dopamine within the synaptic vesicle by dopamine hydroxylase, and it is the only neurotransmitter synthesized from within the vesicle itself.

Further Reading: Psarros. The Definitive Neurosurgical Board Review, page 3.

Greenstein B, Greenstein A. Color Atlas of Neuroscience, 2000.

Citow, Macdonald, Refai. Comprehensive Neurosurgery Board Review, 2nd edition, 2010, physiology section.

50.

C Tyrosine hydroxylase

NE synthesis begins with the amino acid tyrosine. It is converted into L-DOPA by tyrosine hydroxylase, the rate-limiting step. Next, aromatic amino acid decarboxylase synthesizes dopamine from L-DOPA, and then dopamine is taken up into synaptic vesicles where dopamine hydroxylase synthesizes NE from dopamine.

Further Reading: Psarros. The Definitive Neurosurgical Board Review, page 3.

Greenstein B, Greenstein A. Color Atlas of Neuroscience, 2000.

Citow, Macdonald, Refai. Comprehensive Neurosurgery Board Review, 2nd edition, 2010, physiology section.

12 Neuropathology

1.

B EGFR amplification

The pathology slide demonstrates evidence of glioblastoma, notable for pseudopalisading necrosis. GBM often demonstrates amplification of EGFR, and this can also be a reason for tumor transition from anaplastic astrocytoma to GBM.

Further Reading: Psaaros. The Definitive Neurosurgical Board Review, page 126.

Bernstein, Berger. Neuro-Oncology - The Essentials, 3rd edition, 2015, malignant gliomas.

2.

C Loss of sex chromosome

The pathology slide demonstrates an anaplastic astrocytoma, a WHO grade III glioma. Genetic mutations include P53 mutations and loss of sex chromosome. They often demonstrate GFAP positivity and occasionally S-100 positivity.

Further Reading: Psaaros. The Definitive Neurosurgical Board Review, page 126.

Bernstein, Berger. Neuro-Oncology - The Essentials, 3rd edition, 2015, pathology and molecular classification.

3.

B IDH mutant

IDH mutations are becoming important for both glioma identification/characterization as well as prognostication. IDH mutations in primary GBM are very rare. IDH mutations are much more commonly found in WHO grade II-III lesions. If a GBM is found to have IDH mutations, it is likely that it transformed from a lower grade glial neoplasm.

Further Reading: Cohen et al. IDH1 and IDH2 Mutations in Glioma. 2013.

Bernstein, Berger. Neuro-Oncology - The Essentials, 3rd edition, 2015, low grade gliomas.

4.

A Prominent Rosenthal fibers

This MRI is suggestive of a pilocytic astrocytoma, given the cystic component with an enhancing nodule. Histologically, these tumors demonstrate parallel arrangement of bipolar astrocytes with Rosenthal fibers and eosinophilic granular bodies.

Further Reading: Psaaros. The Definitive Neurosurgical Board Review, page 127.

Bernstein, Berger. Neuro-Oncology - The Essentials, 3rd edition, 2015, pilocytic astrocytoma and other indolent tumors.

5.

C Seizures

This pathology slide demonstrates eosinophilic granular bodies and a "storiform" pattern of cellular organization. This is common in pleomorphic xanthoastrocytoma. Intense reticulin staining can also be observed. These tumors often develop in the temporal lobe, have cystic components and present with seizures.

Further Reading: Psaaros. The Definitive Neurosurgical Board Review, page 127.

Bernstein, Berger. Neuro-Oncology - The Essentials, 3rd edition, 2015, perioperative management.

6.

A Cortical malformations

This pathology slide demonstrates gemistocytic type cells with a large eosinophilic cytoplasm and a large eccentric nucleus seen in subependymal giant cell astrocytomas. These tumors are seen in tuberous sclerosis, where cortical tubers can also be seen.

Further Reading: Psaaros. The Definitive Neurosurgical Board Review, page 128.

Bernstein, Berger. Neuro-Oncology - The Essentials, 3rd edition, 2015, familial tumor syndromes.

7.

D 1p/19q co-deletion

This pathology slide demonstrates classic "fried-egg" appearance of oligodendrogliomas. These tumors often demonstrate 1p/19q co-deletion, and this finding is helpful for both therapeutic and prognostic applications.

Further Reading: Psaaros. The Definitive Neurosurgical Board Review, page 128.

Bernstein, Berger. Neuro-Oncology - The Essentials, 3rd edition, 2015, pathology and molecular classification.

8.

B EMA positivity

This pathology slide demonstrates classic periventricular pseudorosettes and uniform cells with variable nuclear : cytoplasmic ratio commonly seen in ependymoma. These tumors often present in the ventricle, and are found to be GFAP, PTAH and EMA positive.

Further Reading: Psaaros. The Definitive Neurosurgical Board Review, page 128.

Bernstein, Berger. Neuro-Oncology - The Essentials, 3rd edition, 2015, pathology and molecular classification.

9.

D Lack of gadolinium enhancement on MRI

This pathology slide demonstrates classic subependymoma, showing small groups of cells with scant cytoplasm in a fibrillary background (islands of blue in a sea of pink). These tumors are often slow growing and can be completely asymptomatic, but due to their location in the 4th ventricle in most adults, they can present with hydrocephalus. On MRI, they classically are an intraventricular lesion that does not demonstrate enhancement with gadolinium.

Further Reading: Bernstein, Berger. Neuro-Oncology - The Essentials, 3rd edition, 2015, intraventricular tumors.

Psaaros. The Definitive Neurosurgical Board Review, page 128.

10.

D Ganglioglioma

This slide demonstrates ganglioglioma, which is often seen to have binucleate cells (ganglion cells) with eosinophilic granular bodies. It is often seen in children at 5-6 years of age and present often with intractable seizures.

Further Reading: Psaaros. The Definitive Neurosurgical Board Review, page 128.

Bernstein, Berger. Neuro-Oncology - The Essentials, 3rd edition, 2015, pilocytic astrocytomas and other indolent tumors.

11.

A Attached to septum pellucidum

This slide demonstrates a central neurocytoma, with homogenous cells with round nuclei on a fibrillary background. These tumors are found within the lateral ventricle attached to the septum pellucidum.

Further Reading: Psaaros. The Definitive Neurosurgical Board Review, page 129.

Bernstein, Berger. Neuro-Oncology - The Essentials, 3rd edition, 2015, Intraventricular tumors.

12.

B Steroids

This slide demonstrates a cellular proliferation around small vascular channels/arterioles. This is highly suggestive of CNS lymphoma, and initial treatment can be carried out with steroids.

Bernstein, Berger. Neuro-Oncology - The Essentials, 3rd edition, 2015, primary central nervous system lymphoma.

13.

D Arachnoid cap cells

This slide demonstrates a classic meningioma. These tumors develop from arachnoid cap cells.

Further Reading: Psaaros. The Definitive Neurosurgical Board Review, page 131.

Bernstein, Berger. Neuro-Oncology - The Essentials, 3rd edition, 2015, meningiomas

14.

B Psammomatous

This slide demonstrates a classic psammomatous meningioma. While multiple subtypes of meninigomas may demonstrate psammoma bodies, when there is a high concentration of these structures, the overall morphology is likely a psammomatous meningoma.

Further Reading: Psaaros. The Definitive Neurosurgical Board Review, page 131.

Bernstein, Berger. Neuro-Oncology - The Essentials, 3rd edition, 2015, meningiomas.

15.

B Loss of chromosome 22

The slide demonstrates a meningioma. The most common genetic malformation in meningioma is loss of chromosome 22.

Further Reading: Psaaros. The Definitive Neurosurgical Board Review, page 131.

Bernstein, Berger. Neuro-Oncology - The Essentials, 3rd edition, 2015, meningiomas.

16.

C Rhabdoid

Papillary, rhabdoid and anaplastic meningiomas are considered WHO grade III. Atypical and chordoid meningomas are considered WHO grade II, and all others are considered WHO grade I.

Further Reading: Psaaros. The Definitive Neurosurgical Board Review, page 131.

Bernstein, Berger. Neuro-Oncology - The Essentials, 3rd edition, 2015, meningiomas.

17.

A Vimentin

Meningiomas often have vimentin, EMA and occasionally S-100 positivity.

Further Reading: Psaaros. The Definitive Neurosurgical Board Review, page 131.

Bernstein, Berger. Neuro-Oncology - The Essentials, 3rd edition, 2015, meningiomas.

18.

D Pineal

The tumor type depicted is a pineoblastoma. It is a poorly differentiated cancer of embryonal origin that demonstrates sheets of blue cells forming classic Flexner-Wintersteiner rosettes, pictured here. These are rosettes formed around cellular extensions rather than a blood vessel.

Further Reading: Psaaros. The Definitive Neurosurgical Board Review.

Bernstein, Berger. Neuro-Oncology - The Essentials, 3rd edition, 2015, pineal region tumors.

19.

B gsp

The patient has signs of acromegaly, suggestive of a GH-secreting pituitary adenoma. 40% of GH-secreting adenomas exhibit a mutation of gsp.

Further Reading: Psaaros. The Definitive Neurosurgical Board Review, page 131.

Bernstein, Berger. Neuro-Oncology - The Essentials, 3rd edition, 2015, pituitary tumors.

20.

A GH

Large, non-functioning pituitary adenomas can cause pituitary failure due to compression of the gland. GH is often the first peptide to be noticeably diminished in this setting.

Further Reading: Psaaros. The Definitive Neurosurgical Board Review, page 132.

Bernstein, Berger. Neuro-Oncology - The Essentials, 3rd edition, 2015, pituitary tumors.

21.

C Papillary cranyiopharyngioma

The histologic slide demonstrates a papillary craniopharyngioma, the subtype more commonly found in adults. Adamantinomatous subtypes exhibit cholesterol clefts and scattered calcification.

Further Reading: Psaaros. The Definitive Neurosurgical Board Review, page 132.

Bernstein, Berger. Neuro-Oncology - The Essentials, 3rd edition, 2015, craniopharyngioma.

22.

B EMA negative

This slide demonstrates a hemangiopericytoma, with classic staghorn vessels. While both meningiomas and HPCs stain positive for vimentin, HPCs are EMA negative while meningiomas are EMA positive.

Further Reading: Psaaros. The Definitive Neurosurgical Board Review, page 132.

Bernstein, Berger. Neuro-Oncology - The Essentials, 3rd edition, 2015, intraventricular tumors.

23.

A Colloid cyst

This slide demonstrates a colloid cyst. The patient presented with headaches and likely low grade hydrocephalus. These lesions present within the third ventricle at the level of the foramen of Monro. They can transiently obstruct CSF flow leading to hydrocephalus. Histologically, they demonstrate a fibrous capsule with an inner epithelial layer and proteinaceous material within the cyst itself.

Further Reading: Psaaros. The Definitive Neurosurgical Board Review, page 132.

Bernstein, Berger. Neuro-Oncology - The Essentials, 3rd edition, 2015, endoscopic approaches.

24.

B Pars intermedia

This slide demonstrates a Rathke's cleft cyst, as evident by the cleft as well as normal surrounding pituitary tissue. These masses arise from the pars intermedia of the pituitary gland.

Further Reading: Psaaros. The Definitive Neurosurgical Board Review, page 132.

Bernstein, Berger. Neuro-Oncology - The Essentials, 3rd edition, 2015, craniopharyngiomas.

25.

B Floor of the 4th ventricle

The slide demonstrates perivascular pseudorosettes, columnar cells surrounding blood vessels. This is a classic finding for ependymoma, which is thought to arise from the floor of the 4th ventricle. Often times these tumors present with nausea compared to subependymomas.

Further Reading: Psaaros. The Definitive Neurosurgical Board Review, page 128.

Bernstein, Berger. Neuro-Oncology - The Essentials, 3rd edition, 2015, pediatric posterior fossa tumors.

26.

B Vimentin

This slide demonstrates an ependymoma, classic with perivascular pseudorosettes. Ependymomas often have a loss of chromosome 22 and exhibit GFAP, PTAH and EMA positivity.

Further Reading: Psaaros. The Definitive Neurosurgical Board Review, page 128.

Bernstein, Berger. Neuro-Oncology - The Essentials, 3rd edition, 2015, pediatric posterior fossa tumors.

27.

A Subependymoma

This patient had a subependymoma resected. These masses classically do not enhance on MRI, and pathology demonstrates "islands of blue in a sea of pink."

Further Reading: Psaaros. The Definitive Neurosurgical Board Review, page 128.

Bernstein, Berger. Neuro-Oncology - The Essentials, 3rd edition, 2015, intraventricular tumors.

28.

C Paraganglioma

The slide demonstrates a paraganglioma, with evidence of capillary networks and nests of chief cells. These lesions can secrete bioactive amines.

Further Reading: Psaaros. The Definitive Neurosurgical Board Review, page 129.

Bernstein, Berger. Neuro-Oncology - The Essentials, 3rd edition, 2015, skull base meningiomas and other tumors.

29.

D Lhermitte-Duclos disease

This MRI demonstrates findings consistent with Lhermitte-Duclos disease, with evidence of hypertrophic cerebellar folia.

Further Reading: Psaaros. The Definitive Neurosurgical Board Review, page 129.

Bernstein, Berger. Neuro-Oncology - The Essentials, 3rd edition, 2015, pilocytic astrocytomas and other indolent tumors.

30.

C PTEN

This MRI demonstrates findings consistent with Lhermitte-Duclos disease, with evidence of hypertrophic cerebellar folia. This finding can be seen in patients with Cowden's syndrome, often caused by a mutation in PTEN.

Further Reading: Psaaros. The Definitive Neurosurgical Board Review, page 129.

Bernstein, Berger. Neuro-Oncology - The Essentials, 3rd edition, 2015, pilocytic astrocytomas and other indolent tumors.

31.

B Choroid plexus papilloma

The slide demonstrates a choroid plexus papilloma, which often arises from the 4th ventricle in adults. They exhibit columnar epithelium in papillary extensions with an interior fibrovascular region.

Further Reading: Psaaros. The Definitive Neurosurgical Board Review, page 130.

Bernstein, Berger. Neuro-Oncology - The Essentials, 3rd edition, 2015, intraventricular tumors.

32.

A P53

The slide demonstrates a choroid plexus papilloma, which has been shown to be associated with Li-Fraumeni syndrome, a syndrome caused by germline mutations in P53. CPPs are vimentin, GFAP and S100 positive.

Further Reading: Psaaros. The Definitive Neurosurgical Board Review, page 130.

Bernstein, Berger. Neuro-Oncology - The Essentials, 3rd edition, 2015, intraventricular tumors.

33.

A Antoni A

This slide demonstrates a schwanomma with two distinct histologic areas. The black arrow is located within an area with prominent fascicles of spindle shaped cells, indicative of an Antoni-A area.

Further Reading: Psaaros. The Definitive Neurosurgical Board Review, page 130.

Bernstein, Berger. Neuro-Oncology - The Essentials, 3rd edition, 2015, schwannomas.

34.

C Verocay body

This slide demonstrates a schwanomma and prominently displays a Verocay body, classically described as "sequential nuclear palisading."

Further Reading: Psaaros. The Definitive Neurosurgical Board Review, page 130.

Bernstein, Berger. Neuro-Oncology - The Essentials, 3rd edition, 2015, schwannomas.

35.

C Endoneurium

Neurofibromas are distinct from schwannomas and are thought to arise from the endoneurium of peripheral nerves.

Further Reading: Psaaros. The Definitive Neurosurgical Board Review, page 130.

Bernstein, Berger. Neuro-Oncology - The Essentials, 3rd edition, 2015, spinal column tumors.

36.

D Neurofibroma

This slide demonstrates a neurofibroma, characterized by spindle-cells in a wavy pattern with large amounts of collagen and a myxoid background. They are often seen in NF1.

Further Reading: Psaaros. The Definitive Neurosurgical Board Review, page 130.

Bernstein, Berger. Neuro-Oncology - The Essentials, 3rd edition, 2015, spinal column tumors.

37.

A Vimentin

This slide demonstrates a neurofibroma, characterized by spindle-cells in a wavy pattern with large amounts of collagen and a myxoid background. Classically they stain positive for S-100.

Further Reading: Psaaros. The Definitive Neurosurgical Board Review, page 130.

Bernstein, Berger. Neuro-Oncology - The Essentials, 3rd edition, 2015, spinal column tumors.

38.

B MPNST

This slide demonstrates an MPNST, with the "storiform cellular pattern, prominent mitoses in a fascicular pattern." Necrosis can also be seen on histology of MPNSTs.

Further Reading: Psaaros. The Definitive Neurosurgical Board Review, page 131.

Bernstein, Berger. Neuro-Oncology - The Essentials, 3rd edition, 2015, peripheral nerve tumors and tumor-like conditions.

39.

A 3

This slide demonstrates a hemangioblastoma, with a dense network of vascular channels and lipid containing interstitial cells. These tumors are associated with von-Hippel Lindau syndrome, characterized by a mutation on chromosome 3.

Further Reading: Psaaros. The Definitive Neurosurgical Board Review, page 132.

Bernstein, Berger. Neuro-Oncology - The Essentials, 3rd edition, 2015, familial tumor syndromes.

40.

C Epidermoid cyst

This slide demonstrates an epidermoid cyst, characterized by stratified squamous epithelium and significant keratin within the center.

Further Reading: Psaaros. The Definitive Neurosurgical Board Review, page 132.

Bernstein, Berger. Neuro-Oncology - The Essentials, 3rd edition, 2015, skull base meningiomas and other tumors.

41.

D Chordoma

This slide demonstrates a chordoma, with "groups of cells with vacuolated cytoplasm" known as (physaliphorous cells). Glycogen deposits can also be seen. These tumors are locally aggressive, often present within the clivus or sacrum, and originate from remnants of the notochord.

Further Reading: Psaaros. The Definitive Neurosurgical Board Review, page 133.

Bernstein, Berger. Neuro-Oncology - The Essentials, 3rd edition, 2015, skull base meningiomas and other tumors.

42.

C Dysembryoplastic neuroepithelial tumor

This slide demonstrates a DNET, and the history is helpful as well. DNETs occur most commonly in the temporal lobe and can be associated with refractory epilepsy. Histologically, there are multiple mucin containing cysts with glial nodules. These masses are synaptophysin positive and neurofilament protein positive.

Further Reading: Psaaros. The Definitive Neurosurgical Board Review, page 129.

Bernstein, Berger. Neuro-Oncology - The Essentials, 3rd edition, 2015, pediatric supratentorial tumors.

43.

D Group 5

This slide demonstrates findings consistent with medulloblastoma, including multiple, round, blue cells with scant cytoplasm. Occasional Homer-Wright rosettes (true rosette without central lumen or blood vessel) can be seen. There are 4 molecular subtypes of medulloblastoma, including Wnt, SHH, Group 3 and Group 4.

Further Reading: Psaaros. The Definitive Neurosurgical Board Review, page 129.

Bernstein, Berger. Neuro-Oncology - The Essentials, 3rd edition, 2015, pediatric posterior fossa tumors.

44.

B External granular layer of the cerebellum

This slide demonstrates findings consistent with medulloblastoma, and these tumors are though to arise from the roof of the 4th ventricle, specifically the granular layer of the cerebellum. This differentiates their origin from ependymomas of the 4th ventricle.

Further Reading: Psaaros. The Definitive Neurosurgical Board Review, page 129.

Bernstein, Berger. Neuro-Oncology - The Essentials, 3rd edition, 2015, pediatric posterior fossa tumors.

45.

A Placental alkaline phosphatase

This slide demonstrates findings consistent with germinoma, including "round neoplastic cells with prominent clear cytoplasm and large nuclei, occasionally with associated inflammation." CSF markers are important in pediatric suprasellar masses, and an elevated placental alkaline phosphatase can make the diagnosis of germinoma.

Further Reading: Psaaros. The Definitive Neurosurgical Board Review, page 130.

Bernstein, Berger. Neuro-Oncology - The Essentials, 3rd edition, 2015, molecular markers and pathways in brain tumorigenesis.

46.

B B-HCG

This slide demonstrates findings consistent with choriocarcinoma with evidence of syncytiotrophoblastic giant cells. Choriocarcinomas have elevated B-HCG levels.

Further Reading: Psaaros. The Definitive Neurosurgical Board Review, page 130.

Bernstein, Berger. Neuro-Oncology - The Essentials, 3rd edition, 2015, pineal region tumors.

47.

C AFP

This slide demonstrates findings consistent with a yolk sac tumor, with prominent schiller Duval bodies. Yolk-sac tumors are strongly positive for AFP on CSF analysis.

Further Reading: Psaaros. The Definitive Neurosurgical Board Review, page 130.

Bernstein, Berger. Neuro-Oncology - The Essentials, 3rd edition, 2015, pineal region tumors.

48.

A Mature teratoma

This slide demonstrates findings consistent with a mature teratoma, a cystic lesion that contains tissue from ectodermal, endodermal and mesodermal origin. CSF is often negative for aberrations in markers for mature teratomas.

Further Reading: Psaaros. The Definitive Neurosurgical Board Review, page 130.

Bernstein, Berger. Neuro-Oncology - The Essentials, 3rd edition, 2015, molecular markers and pathways in brain tumorigenesis.

49.

A Wnt

This slide demonstrates findings consistent with medulloblastoma, of which there are 4 subtypes, SHH, Wnt, Group 3 and Group 4. With current therapeutics, the Wnt subtype his the longest overall survival, followed by SHH, followed by Group 3/4 tumors.

Further Reading: Bernstein, Berger. Neuro-Oncology - The Essentials, 3rd edition, 2015, pediatric posterior fossa tumors.

50.

B Dermoid cyst

This slide demonstrates findings consistent with a dermoid cyst, containing sebacious glands and keratin. Dermoid cysts are usually found in the midline.

Further Reading: Bernstein, Berger. Neuro-Oncology - The Essentials, 3rd edition, 2015, skull base meningiomas and other tumors.

13 Neuroimaging

1.

C Glioma

This MR spectroscopy (MRS) image demonstrates an area of abnormality in the left insula. On MRS, the choline peak is much higher than the N-acetylaspartate (NAA) or creatine peak. This is suggestive of glioma.

Further Reading: Jain, Essig. Brain Tumor Imaging, 2015, metabolic imaging: MR spectroscopy.

2.

B Infarction

MRS can be used to determine what an abnormality may be when seen on MRI. The classic choline peak is suggestive of glioma. When the lactate peak is elevated, ischemic stroke is suggested, given that the brain has switched over to anaerobic metabolism.

Further Reading: Jain, Essig. Brain Tumor Imaging, 2015, metabolic imaging: MR spectroscopy.

3.

D Radiation necrosis

MRS can be difficult to determine the difference between radiation necrosis and recurrent glioma. However, in recurrent glioma, a choline peak would be suggested, while in radiation necrosis, a significant NAA peak can be seen.

Further Reading: Jain, Essig. Brain Tumor Imaging, 2015, metabolic imaging: MR spectroscopy.

4.

D IDH-1 wild type

This MRI is suggestive of a glioblastoma (GBM), based on ring enhancement of a "butterfly" lesion. Most primary GBMs are IDH-1 wild type and, when found to be IDH-1 mutant, may be suggestive of a malignant transformation from a lower grade glioma.

Further Reading: Bernstein, Berger. Neuro-Oncology: The Essentials, 3rd edition, 2015, malignant gliomas.

5.

A Glioblastoma

This MRI demonstrates evidence of a malignant GBM.

Further Reading: Bernstein, Berger. Neuro-Oncology: The Essentials, 3rd edition, 2015, malignant gliomas.

6.

B Meningioma

This MRI demonstrates a classic appearance of a meningioma with associated dural tails.

Further Reading: Bernstein, Berger. Neuro-Oncology: The Essentials, 3rd edition, 2015, meningiomas.

7.

B WHO grade II

This MRI demonstrates a classic appearance of a meningioma with associated dural tails. If pathology determined this to be chordoid type, it would make it an atypical, or WHO grade II lesion.

Further Reading: Bernstein, Berger. Neuro-Oncology: The Essentials, 3rd edition, 2015, meningiomas.

8.

C Hemangiopericytoma

This MRI demonstrates an invasive lesion that appears to be associated with the meninges. It has a look of a meningioma, but in this case was a hemangiopericytoma. When these tumors are based in the meninges, they can closely resemble meningiomas, but may appear much more vascular and may have more associated cerebral edema.

Further Reading: Bernstein, Berger. Neuro-Oncology: The Essentials, 3rd edition, 2015, intraventricular tumors.

9.

B Gray–white matter junction

This MRI demonstrates evidence of multiple metastatic lesions. These lesions most often are located at the gray–white matter junction as this is the level of the small capillaries that tend to filter out cells as they metastasize.

Further Reading: Bernstein, Berger. Neuro-Oncology: The Essentials, 3rd edition, 2015, metastatic brain tumors.

10.

A Skin

This MRI demonstrates a cerebral metastasis with significant edema and a fluid–fluid level within the mass suggestive of hemorrhage. The hemorrhagic nature of this mass makes it most likely to be melanoma out of the choices listed above. Renal cell metastases are also known to hemorrhage.

Further Reading: Bernstein, Berger. Neuro-Oncology: The Essentials, 3rd edition, 2015, metastatic brain tumors.

11.

D 22

This MRI demonstrates bilateral vestibular schwannomas. This is very common in patients with NF2, caused by a chromosomal abnormality on chromosome 22.

Further Reading: Bernstein, Berger. Neuro-Oncology: The Essentials, 3rd edition, 2015, vestibular schwannomas.

12.

B Epidermoid cyst

This diffusion-weighted MRI demonstrates a cerebellopontine (CP) angle mass that is bright on diffusion images. This finding is consistent with an epidermoid cyst of the CP angle. The diffusion scans are important to evaluate with CP angle masses to rule out epidermoid cysts, as they are the mass in this region that are bright on diffusion.

Further Reading: Bernstein, Berger. Neuro-Oncology: The Essentials, 3rd edition, 2015, skull base meningiomas and other tumors.

13.

D Ependymoma

This gadolinium-enhanced MRI demonstrates an expansile mass with heterogenous enhancement within the fourth ventricle. It also extends laterally through the foramen of Luschka. This, along with the history of nausea at presentation, makes ependymoma the most likely diagnosis. Ependymomas are known to extend laterally, enhance, and cause nausea at presentation. There is also an association between these tumors and NF2.

Further Reading: Bernstein, Berger. Neuro-Oncology: The Essentials, 3rd edition, 2015, pediatric posterior fossa tumors.

14.

B Luschka

This gadolinium-enhanced MRI demonstrates an expansile mass with heterogenous enhancement within the fourth ventricle. It also extends laterally through the foramen of Luschka. This, along with the history of nausea at presentation, makes ependymoma the most likely diagnosis. Ependymomas are known to extend laterally, enhance, and cause nausea at presentation. There is also an association between these tumors and NF2.

Further Reading: Bernstein, Berger. Neuro-Oncology: The Essentials, 3rd edition, 2015, pediatric posterior fossa tumors.

15.

B Subependymoma

This gadolinium-enhanced MRI demonstrates a mass within the fourth ventricle that does not enhance. This is a classic picture for a subependymoma. While ependymomas can also present in the fourth ventricle, they generally have a heterogenous enhancement pattern.

Further Reading: Bernstein, Berger. Neuro-Oncology: The Essentials, 3rd edition, 2015, intraventricular tumors.

16.

D PICA aneurysm

This T2 sequence axial MRI demonstrates a large mass in the posterior fossa. There is T2 hypointensity within the mass in a somewhat layered form. Given the location and the appearance on T2, this should be concerning for a posterior fossa aneurysm.

Further Reading: Spetzler, Kalani, Nakaji. Neurovascular Surgery, 2nd edition, 2015, surgical therapies for vertebral artery and posterior inferior cerebellar artery aneurysms.

17.

C Cavernous malformation

These MRI sequences demonstrate a mass within the brainstem consistent with a cavernous malformation. Cavernomas often appear very dark on gradient-echo (GRE) sequences owing to bleeding events.

Further Reading: Spetzler, Kalani, Nakaji. Neurovascular Surgery, 2nd edition, 2015, cavernous malformations: natural history, epidemiology, presentation, and treatment options.

18.

D Persistent trigeminal artery

This lateral DSA of the ICA demonstrates filling of both the ICA and posterior circulation simultaneously. There is a persistent trigeminal artery connecting the ICA to the basilar artery. It is the most common persistent connection between the ICA and basilar systems. A fetal PCA would be an enlarged posterior communicating artery with an absent ipsilateral P1 segment.

Further Reading: Spetzler, Kalani, Nakaji. Neurovascular Surgery, 2nd edition, 2015, cranial vascular anatomy of the posterior circulation.

19.

B Carotid-ophthalmic aneurysm

This DSA of the ICA demonstrates an aneurysm of the ophthalmic segment of the ICA. It is superiorly projecting, which makes it most likely a carotid ophthalmic aneurysm. Superior hypophyseal aneurysms can arise in the same location, but tend to project inferomedially rather than superolaterally.

Further Reading: Spetzler, Kalani, Nakaji. Neurovascular Surgery, 2nd edition, 2015, endovascular treatment of carotid-ophthalmic aneurysms.

20.

B Intracranial/extradural

This angiogram of the ICA demonstrates a petrous/cavernous segment fusiform aneurysm, making it intracranial, but extradural. This makes these aneurysms much more stable and in some cases, they do not require treatment (mainly for stable cavernous segment aneurysms). When they rupture, a direct/indirect CC fistula can occur and patients can present with paralysis of the eye, as well as chemosis, proptosis, and venous congestion on the ipsilateral eye.

Further Reading: Spetzler, Kalani, Nakaji. Neurovascular Surgery, 2nd edition, 2015, endovascular therapies for aneurysms of the internal carotid artery.

21.

B Anastomotic vein of Labbé

The arrows in this magnetic resonance venography (MRV) are demonstrating the inferior anastomotic vein (of Labbé). It is an important structure as damage the vein of Labbé can lead to venous infarction of the temporal lobe.

Further Reading: Spetzler, Kalani, Nakaji. Neurovascular Surgery, 2nd edition, 2015, cranial venous anatomy.

22.

C Size greater than 1.0 cm

This coronal MRI demonstrates a pituitary macroadenoma given that the size of the adenoma is greater than 1.0 cm.

Further Reading: Schwartz, Anand. Endoscopic Pituitary Surgery, 2012, radiographic evaluation of pituitary tumors.

23.

C Tuberculum meningioma

This enhanced MRI demonstrates a suprasellar mass. It is most consistent with a tuberculum meningioma due to the dural tail.

Further Reading: Di Ieva, Lee, Cusimano. Handbook of Skull Base Surgery, 2016, endoscopic transsphenoidal approaches.

24.

A Neurofibromatosis type 1 (NF1)

This MRI demonstrates enlargement of the optic nerve in a pediatric patient consistent with an optic pathway glioma. These tumors are highly associated with neurofibromatosis type 1 (NF1).

Further Reading: Bernstein, Berger. Neuro-Oncology: The Essentials, 3rd edition, 2015, pediatric supratentorial tumors.

25.

C 9

This MRI demonstrates a homogenously enhancing mass at the level of the foramen of Monro most consistent with a subependymal giant cell astrocytoma. These tumors are found in tuberous sclerosis, which can be caused by a mutation in tuberous sclerosis 1 (TSC1) on chromosome 9.

Further Reading: Bernstein, Berger. Neuro-Oncology: The Essentials, 3rd edition, 2015, familial tumor syndromes.

26.

D Internal cerebral veins

In this coronal MRI, the white arrowheads are pointing to the paired internal cerebral veins within the third ventricle.

Further Reading: Bernstein, Berger. Neuro-Oncology: The Essentials, 3rd edition, 2015, cranial venous anatomy.

27.

D Hippocampus

This coronal MRI is T2 weighted, and number 18 demonstrates the hippocampal formation. It is important to identify the hippocampus, especially in patients in whom there is concern for mesial temporal sclerosis and seizures.

Further Reading: Cataltepe, Jallo. Pediatric Epilepsy Surgery, 2010, resective surgical techniques in temporal lobe epilepsy: transsylvian selective amygdalohippocampectomy.

28.

C Posterior reversible encephalopathy syndrome

This MRI demonstrates T2 hyperintensities within the parieto-occipital lobes bilaterally. This, associated with seizures on presentation, is classic for posterior reversible encephalopathy syndrome (PRES).

Further Reading: Harbaugh, Shaffrey, Couldwell, Berger. Neurosurgery Knowledge Update, 2015, posterior reversible encephalopathy syndrome.

29.

A Start acyclovir

This MRI demonstrates hyperintensities within the anterior temporal lobes bilaterally. In the setting of a rapidly declining patient with seizures, herpes encephalitis should be strongly considered and acyclovir should be initiated.

Further Reading: Hall, Kim. Neurosurgical Infectious Disease, 2014, radiology of central nervous system infections.

30.

B Neurocysticercosis

This MRI demonstrates multiple lesions within the cerebrum. Each lesion demonstrates T2 hyperintensities within the central core as well as a hypointense region within the cyst, the classic "cyst with a dot sign." This MRI is consistent with neurocysticercosis.

Further Reading: Hall, Kim. Neurosurgical Infectious Disease, 2014, radiology of central nervous system infections.

31.

B CMV encephalitis

This CT scan demonstrates diffuse periventricular calcifications and hydrocephalus, findings associated with CMV encephalitis in the pediatric population.

Further Reading: Hall, Kim. Neurosurgical Infectious Disease, 2014, microbiological diagnosis of central nervous system infections.

32.

A Multiple sclerosis

This MRI demonstrates the classic periventricular hyperintensities, "Dawnson's fingers" associated with multiple sclerosis. The intermittent nature of the deficits helps point toward the diagnosis of MS.

Further Reading: Forsting, Jansen. MR Neuroimaging: Brain, Spine, Peripheral Nerves, 2017, multiple sclerosis and related diseases.

33.

C Tumefactive multiple sclerosis

This MRI demonstrates an acute, fulminant demyelinating process causing severe mass effect consistent with tumefactive MS. There is incomplete ring enhancement and decreased perfusion to the region, making GBM less likely.

Further Reading: Forsting, Jansen. MR Neuroimaging: Brain, Spine, Peripheral Nerves, 2017, multiple sclerosis and related diseases.

34.

A Very long chain fatty acid synthesis

This MRI demonstrates white matter edema that appears to spare the subcortical U-fibers. This can be seen in X-linked adrenoleukodystrophy, which is caused by an abnormality in very long chain fatty acid synthesis.

Further Reading: Forsting, Jansen. MR Neuroimaging: Brain, Spine, Peripheral Nerves, 2017, metabolic disorders.

35.

B Cerebral abscess

This CT demonstrates a cortical ring enhancing mass with significant surrounding edema. Given the clinical history, cerebral abscess should be high on the differential. Metastatic lesions can cause this much edema, but GBM often does not present with this much perilesional edema.

Further Reading: Forsting, Jansen. MR Neuroimaging: Brain, Spine, Peripheral Nerves, 2017, infections.

36.

A *Streptococcus milleri*

This MRI demonstrates a cortical ring enhancing mass with significant surrounding edema.

Given the clinical history, cerebral abscess should be high on the differential. The most common isolate from primary cerebral abscesses listed here is *Streptococcus milleri*.

Further Reading: Forsting, Jansen. MR Neuroimaging: Brain, Spine, Peripheral Nerves, 2017, infections.

37.

D Lymphocytic hypophysitis

This sagittal MRI demonstrates an enlarged pituitary gland as well as an enlarged infundibular stalk, both of which enhance with contrast. Given the female gender and history of recent pregnancy, lymphocytic hypophysitis should be strongly considered. This condition is often self-limited.

Further Reading: Forsting, Jansen. MR Neuroimaging: Brain, Spine, Peripheral Nerves, 2017, brain tumors.

38.

D Give hydrocortisone

This MRI demonstrates pituitary hemorrhage, and in this patient, consistent with Sheehan's syndrome, a pituitary infarction caused by large-volume blood loss during delivery. After necrosis of the pituitary gland, hemorrhage can occur. These patients can decompensate quickly due to further hypotension given a complete lack of cortisol. Hydrocortisone should be given immediately and, next, consideration of pituitary decompression should be considered to save vision.

Further Reading: Forsting, Jansen. MR Neuroimaging: Brain, Spine, Peripheral Nerves, 2017, brain tumors.

39.

C Neurosarcoidosis

This skull base MRI demonstrates diffuse, homogenous enhancement of cranial nerves, and the leptomeninges. This finding, with cranial neuropathies, can be consistent with neurosarcoidosis.

Further Reading: Forsting, Jansen. MR Neuroimaging: Brain, Spine, Peripheral Nerves, 2017, brain tumors.

40.

B Dopamine

This MRI demonstrates the substantia nigra, which uses dopamine as its primary neurotransmitter.

Further Reading: Forsting, Jansen. MR Neuroimaging: Brain, Spine, Peripheral Nerves, 2017, anatomy.

41.

C Frontotemporal dementia

This MRI demonstrates atrophy of the frontal lobe with sparing of the parietal lobes. These findings, along with socially disruptive behavior and personality changes, are consistent with frontotemporal dementia. This term is becoming antiquated, and behavioral variant FTLD (frontotemporal lobe degeneration) is being used. It has also been termed Pick's disease, but this should refer only to patients with histologically proven Pick's bodies.

Further Reading: Forsting, Jansen. MR Neuroimaging: Brain, Spine, Peripheral Nerves, 2017, degenerative diseases.

42.

A Isointense

Blood products on MRI are highly testable and annoying to memorize. Several mnemonics exist, but consider the classic mnemonic I Be, iDDy, BiDy, BaBy, DooDoo. Hyperacute (< 24 hours) = I B (T1/T2) or T1 isointense and T2 hyperintense. Acute (1–3 days) = DD (T1 dark, T2 dark), early subacute (3–7 days) = BD (T1 bright, T2 dark), late subacute (7–14 days) = BB (T1 bright, T2 bright), chronic (> 14 days) = DD (T1 dark, T2 dark).

Further Reading: Forsting, Jansen. MR Neuroimaging: Brain, Spine, Peripheral Nerves, 2017, vascular diseases.

43.

B Hyperintense

Blood products on MRI are highly testable and annoying to memorize. Several mnemonics exist, but consider the classic mnemonic I Be, iDDy, BiDy, BaBy, DooDoo. Hyperacute (< 24 hours) = I B (T1/T2) or T1 isointense and T2 hyperintense. Acute (1–3 days) = DD (T1 dark, T2 dark), early subacute (3–7 days) = BD (T1 bright, T2 dark), late subacute (7–14 days) = BB (T1 bright, T2 bright), chronic (> 14 days) = DD (T1 dark, T2 dark).

Further Reading: Forsting, Jansen. MR Neuroimaging: Brain, Spine, Peripheral Nerves, 2017, vascular diseases.

44.

C Hypointense

Blood products on MRI are highly testable and annoying to memorize. Several mnemonics exist, but consider the classic mnemonic I Be, iDDy, BiDy, BaBy, DooDoo. Hyperacute (< 24 hours) = I B (T1/T2) or T1 isointense and T2 hyperintense. Acute (1–3 days) = DD (T1 dark, T2 dark), early subacute (3–7 days) = BD (T1 bright, T2 dark), late subacute (7–14 days) = BB (T1 bright, T2 bright), chronic (> 14 days) = DD (T1 dark, T2 dark).

Further Reading: Forsting, Jansen. MR Neuroimaging: Brain, Spine, Peripheral Nerves, 2017, vascular diseases.

45.

C Hypointense

Blood products on MRI are highly testable and annoying to memorize. Several mnemonics exist, but consider the classic mnemonic I Be, iDDy, BiDy, BaBy, DooDoo. Hyperacute (< 24 hours) = I B (T1/T2) or T1 isointense and T2 hyperintense. Acute (1–3 days) = DD (T1 dark, T2 dark), early subacute (3–7 days) = BD (T1 bright, T2 dark), late subacute (7–14 days) = BB (T1 bright, T2 bright), chronic (> 14 days) = DD (T1 dark, T2 dark).

Further Reading: Forsting, Jansen. MR Neuroimaging: Brain, Spine, Peripheral Nerves, 2017, vascular diseases.

46.

B Hyperintense

Blood products on MRI are highly testable and annoying to memorize. Several mnemonics exist, but consider the classic mnemonic I Be, iDDy, BiDy, BaBy, DooDoo. Hyperacute (< 24 hours) = I B (T1/T2) or T1 isointense and T2 hyperintense. Acute (1–3 days) = DD (T1 dark, T2 dark), early subacute (3–7 days) = BD (T1 bright, T2 dark), late subacute (7–14 days) = BB (T1 bright, T2 bright), chronic (> 14 days) = DD (T1 dark, T2 dark).

Further Reading: Forsting, Jansen. MR Neuroimaging: Brain, Spine, Peripheral Nerves, 2017, vascular diseases.

47.

C Hypointense

Blood products on MRI are highly testable and annoying to memorize. Several mnemonics exist, but consider the classic mnemonic I Be, iDDy, BiDy, BaBy, DooDoo. Hyperacute (< 24 hours) = I B (T1/T2) or T1 isointense and T2 hyperintense. Acute (1–3 days) = DD (T1 dark, T2 dark), early subacute (3–7 days) = BD (T1 bright, T2 dark), late subacute (7–14 days) = BB (T1 bright, T2 bright), chronic (> 14 days) = DD (T1 dark, T2 dark).

Further Reading: Forsting, Jansen. MR Neuroimaging: Brain, Spine, Peripheral Nerves, 2017, vascular diseases.

48.

B Hyperintense

Blood products on MRI are highly testable and annoying to memorize. Several mnemonics exist, but consider the classic mnemonic I Be, iDDy, BiDy, BaBy, DooDoo. Hyperacute (< 24 hours) = I B (T1/T2) or T1 isointense and T2 hyperintense. Acute (1–3 days) = DD (T1 dark, T2 dark), early subacute (3–7 days) = BD (T1 bright, T2 dark), late subacute (7–14 days) = BB (T1 bright, T2 bright), chronic (> 14 days) = DD (T1 dark, T2 dark).

Further Reading: Forsting, Jansen. MR Neuroimaging: Brain, Spine, Peripheral Nerves, 2017, vascular diseases.

49.

B Hyperintense

Blood products on MRI are highly testable and annoying to memorize. Several mnemonics exist, but consider the classic mnemonic I Be, iDDy, BiDy, BaBy, DooDoo. Hyperacute (< 24 hours) = I B (T1/T2) or T1 isointense and T2 hyperintense. Acute (1–3 days) = DD (T1 dark, T2 dark), early subacute (3–7 days) = BD (T1 bright, T2 dark), late subacute (7–14 days) = BB (T1 bright, T2 bright), chronic (> 14 days) = DD (T1 dark, T2 dark).

Further Reading: Forsting, Jansen. MR Neuroimaging: Brain, Spine, Peripheral Nerves, 2017, vascular diseases.

50.

C Hypointense

Blood products on MRI are highly testable and annoying to memorize. Several mnemonics exist, but consider the classic mnemonic I Be, iDDy, BiDy, BaBy, DooDoo. Hyperacute (< 24 hours) = I B (T1/T2) or T1 isointense and T2 hyperintense. Acute (1–3 days) = DD (T1 dark, T2 dark), early subacute (3–7 days) = BD (T1 bright, T2 dark), late subacute (7–14 days) = BB (T1 bright, T2 bright), chronic (> 14 days) = DD (T1 dark, T2 dark).

Further Reading: Forsting, Jansen. MR Neuroimaging: Brain, Spine, Peripheral Nerves, 2017, vascular diseases.

14 Fundamental Skills

1.

B 8%

In a normal 70-kg man, approximately 67% of fluid is intracellular and 33% is extracellular. Of the extracellular fluid, a further 25% is interstitial, and the remaining approximately 8% is intravascular.

Further Reading: Siddiqi. Neurosurgical Intensive Care, 2017, page 300.

2.

C Shunt externalization/removal

This patient has evidence of a large pleural effusion on the side where the syringopleural shunt has been placed. In this case, the shunt should be externalized or removed completely. General/thoracic surgery can address the pleural effusion, but further treatment of the syrinx will have to be performed via another approach.

Further Reading: Procedures: Syringopleural Shunting, Thieme eNeurosurgery.

3.

B Pulmonary capillary wedge pressure (PCWP) greater than 18 mm Hg

In patients with cardiogenic pulmonary edema, the PCWP is elevated beyond 18 mm Hg. In acute or adult respiratory distress syndrome (ARDS), the PCWP is less than 18 mm Hg.

4.

B Dobutamine

Of the listed medications, only dobutamine has positive effects in patients with severe ARDS. Its inotropic effects can increase cardiac output and thus oxygen delivery.

Further Reading: Citow, Macdonald, Refai. Comprehensive Neurosurgery Board Review, 2nd edition, 2010, page 503.

5.

A Narrow complex tachycardia

Adenosine briefly interrupts transmission through the His–Purkinje system and causes asystole for several seconds. It can be useful for treating supraventricular tachycardia (a narrow complex tachycardia).

Further Reading: Citow, Macdonald, Refai. Comprehensive Neurosurgery Board Review, 2nd edition, 2010, page 498.

6.

B Lidocaine infusion

This patient has a stable, wide complex tachycardia. She could undergo elective, synchronized cardioversion, or infusion of lidocaine, which can treat wide complex tachycardia. The other options are not reasonable in a stable patient.

Further Reading: Citow, Macdonald, Refai. Comprehensive Neurosurgery Board Review, 2nd edition, 2010, page 498.

7.

D 6

The GCS is a commonly used scale for neurotrauma. Points are assigned for motor, verbal and eye-opening responses. This patient gets 3 points for flexor posturing, 2 points for eye opening to pain, and 1 point for no verbal response.

Further Reading: Siddiqi. Neurosurgical Intensive Care, 2017, pages 3–5.

8.

A Normal physiologic response

This patient is exhibiting hippus, a normal physiologic response where the pupils dilate and contract seemingly randomly. It can also be seen during recovery of oculomotor nerve injury.

Further Reading: Siddiqi. Neurosurgical Intensive Care, 2017, page 14.

9.

C Suprachiasmatic nucleus

This patient is experiencing sundowning, where delirium worsens in the evening and at night. It is thought that this is at least partially due to degeneration of the suprachiasmatic nucleus of the hypothalamus, and dysregulation of melatonin release and the circadian rhythm.

Further Reading: Siddiqi. Neurosurgical Intensive Care, 2017, page 31.

10.

E Gamma

Opioid receptors have four classes, mu, delta, kappa, and N/OFQ. Gamma is not an opioid receptor subtype. There is interest in the kappa receptor as a target for pain medication as it may also have neuroprotective effects in traumatic brain injury.

Further Reading: Siddiqi. Neurosurgical Intensive Care, 2017, page 150.

11.

D 9

Warfarin inhibits vitamin K–dependent factors, including factors II, VII, IX, and X and proteins C and S.

Further Reading: Hamilton, Golfinos, Pineo, Couldwell. Handbook of Bleeding and Coagulation for Neurosurgery, 2015, page 47.

12.

E 24+ hours

IV vitamin K has excellent bioavailability and a rapid onset; however, the vitamin K–dependent coagulation factors have long half-lives, with factor II having a half-life of 65 hours. Therefore, it can take between 24 to 72 hours for IV vitamin K to reverse the INR.

Further Reading: Hamilton, Golfinos, Pineo, Couldwell. Handbook of Bleeding and Coagulation for Neurosurgery, 2015, page 48.

13.

D Xa

Heparin binds to antithrombin, and this combination has a high affinity for factor Xa, inhibiting its function and causing anticoagulation. It is monitored using activated partial thromboplastin time (aPTT).

Further Reading: Hamilton, Golfinos, Pineo, Couldwell. Handbook of Bleeding and Coagulation for Neurosurgery, 2015, page 52.

14.

B Dabigatran

Dabigatran is in the class of direct thrombin inhibitors, which can be used for anticoagulation in patients with HIT. Dabigatran is cleared by the kidney, however, and it should be avoided in patients with renal failure. Argatroban is cleared by the liver, and would be a better choice.

Further Reading: Hamilton, Golfinos, Pineo, Couldwell. Handbook of Bleeding and Coagulation for Neurosurgery, 2015, page 54.

15.

A 30 minutes

The half-life of aspirin is very short, only 30 minutes. It has lasting effects, however, due to the irreversible inhibition of platelets, which survive for 7 days. The effect of aspirin will no longer be evident in most patients by 5 to 7 days after the last dose.

Further Reading: Hamilton, Golfinos, Pineo, Couldwell. Handbook of Bleeding and Coagulation for Neurosurgery, 2015, page 55.

16.

B $P2Y_{12}$ receptor binding inhibiting ADP mediated platelet aggregation (GPIIb/IIIa)

Clopidogrel (plavix) inhibits platelet function by binding to the $P2Y_{12}$ receptor and inhibiting ADP-mediated GPIIb/IIIa complex formation. It is irreversible and its effects last until new platelets are formed.

Further Reading: Hamilton, Golfinos, Pineo, Couldwell. Handbook of Bleeding and Coagulation for Neurosurgery, 2015, page 56.

17.

B 0.5 to 1.0 mL/kg/h

Urine output can be a useful determining factor of overall volume status in the postoperative patient. Often, volume resuscitation is targeted to a urine output of 0.5 to 1.0 mL/kg/h.

Further Reading: Hamilton, Golfinos, Pineo, Couldwell. Handbook of Bleeding and Coagulation for Neurosurgery, 2015, page 89.

18.

A Prothrombin complex concentrates

In this patient with heart failure and a need for immediate reversal, PCCs should be used to decrease the overall fluid volume utilized during resuscitation as to not worsen the heart failure.

Further Reading: Hamilton, Golfinos, Pineo, Couldwell. Handbook of Bleeding and Coagulation for Neurosurgery, 2015, page 49.

19.

C 3 months

For patients with an unprovoked deep vein thrombosis (DVT) who are on anticoagulation, the recommended initial treatment period is 3 months. After 3 months, further imaging will be performed to determine if treatment needs to be extended.

Further Reading: Hamilton, Golfinos, Pineo, Couldwell. Handbook of Bleeding and Coagulation for Neurosurgery, 2015, page 129.

20.

A IV heparin

This patient has evidence of a cerebral venous sinus thrombosis. Regardless of the presence of intracerebral hemorrhage (ICH), this patient should receive IV heparin administration in an attempt to dissolve the clot. The presence of hemorrhage is not a contraindication for heparin.

Further Reading: Hamilton, Golfinos, Pineo, Couldwell. Handbook of Bleeding and Coagulation for Neurosurgery, 2015, page 190.

21.

D 20 mm Hg

It is thought that with a brain tissue partial pressure of oxygen below 20 mm Hg, anaerobic respiration predominates, which can lead to secondary brain injury.

Further Reading: Siddiqi. Neurosurgical Intensive Care, 2017, page 329.

22.

C 8 or less

According to these guidelines, a GCS of 8 or less is considered severe head injury, and these patients should be considered for intubation if there is clinical concern for airway protection

Further Reading: Siddiqi. Neurosurgical Intensive Care, 2017, page 330.

23.

C 90 minutes

Rocuronium is a paralytic agent used for intubation. The duration can be 30 to 90 minutes.

Further Reading: Siddiqi. Neurosurgical Intensive Care, 2017, page 333.

24.

B Increased pH

Hyperventilation increases the pH in the brain due to increased ventilation and blowing off of CO_2. This increase in pH causes vasoconstriction, which can decrease blood volume in the brain and subsequently decrease ICP.

Further Reading: Siddiqi. Neurosurgical Intensive Care, 2017, page 335.

25.

C Pons

This breathing pattern is apneustic breathing, suggestive of destruction to the pons.

Further Reading: Siddiqi. Neurosurgical Intensive Care, 2017, page 340.

26.

C 50 mL/100 g/min

CBF in the normal, healthy adult is thought to be around 50 mL/100 g/min.

Further Reading: Siddiqi. Neurosurgical Intensive Care, 2017, page 424.

27.

E 100 mL/100 g/min

Pediatric patients have elevated cerebral blood flow, and it can be as high as 108 mL/100 g/min and it can stay this elevated through the teenage years.

Further Reading: Siddiqi. Neurosurgical Intensive Care, 2017, page 424.

28.

B Small cell lung cancer

Small cell lung cancer has the ability to form peptide hormones, including antidiuretic hormone (ADH), which can lead to syndrome of inappropriate antidiuretic hormone secretion (SIADH) and hyponatremia.

Further Reading: Bernstein, Berger. Neuro-Oncology: The Essentials, 3rd edition, 2015, page 451.

29.

B CSF antineuronal antibodies

Neuropsychiatric SLE can manifest with multiple symptoms. The diagnosis can be made by testing for ANA in the cerebrospinal fluid (CSF).

Further Reading: Kanekar. Imaging of Neurodegenerative Disorders, 2016, page 221.

30.

B CADASIL

This MRI demonstrates findings classic for cerebral autosomal dominant arteriopathy with subcortical infarcts. This is thought to occur due to regional hypometabolism due to a genetic abnormality on chromosome 19. Patients have a progressive declining course and often die between 50 and 70 years of age.

Further Reading: Kanekar. Imaging of Neurodegenerative Disorders, 2016, page 220.

31.

A Inflammation

This patient has giant cell arteritis, also known as temporal arteritis. Blindness is a feared complication when this condition is left untreated, and it occurs via inflammation and progression of disease to include the ciliary arteries and central retinal artery. When inflamed, they can lead to ischemic optic neuropathy and blindness.

Further Reading: Harbaugh, Shaffrey, Couldwell, Berger. Neurosurgery Knowledge Update, 2015, page 249.

32.

C Prednisone

Giant cell arteritis is an inflammatory vasculitis and blindness can be a complication of this condition. These patients should be treated with prednisone initially.

Further Reading: Harbaugh, Shaffrey, Couldwell, Berger. Neurosurgery Knowledge Update, 2015, page 249.

33.

C 320

Mannitol should no longer be administered in patients who have a serum osmolality of 320 or greater as the risk of ATN increases substantially.

Further Reading: Harbaugh, Shaffrey, Couldwell, Berger. Neurosurgery Knowledge Update, 2015, page 762.

34.

D Calcified cephalohematoma

This CT scan demonstrates evidence of a calcified cephalohematoma, a bleed located between the periosteum and the skull. It becomes bound by suture lines. In the majority of cases, these resolve in 1 to 3 days; however, they can persist and calcify, sometimes requiring surgery.

Further Reading: Harbaugh, Shaffrey, Couldwell, Berger. Neurosurgery Knowledge Update, 2015, page 798.

35.

A Further observation

At this point, the child is stable and more observation should be recommended. The hematoma may continue to resolve over time. Needle aspiration should be avoided unless there is concern for infection due to the risk of iatrogenic infection.

Further Reading: Harbaugh, Shaffrey, Couldwell, Berger. Neurosurgery Knowledge Update, 2015, page 799.

36.

A 5%

Retinal hemorrhages are very common in non-accidental trauma, and very rare in accidental brain trauma, occurring in 5% or less of accidental traumas.

Further Reading: Harbaugh, Shaffrey, Couldwell, Berger. Neurosurgery Knowledge Update, 2015, page 803.

37.

B < 70 minutes

According to current evidence, decompression should be achieved within 70 minutes of the onset of pupillary changes in patients with EDH, highlighting the emergent nature of this condition.

Further Reading: Harbaugh, Shaffrey, Couldwell, Berger. Neurosurgery Knowledge Update, 2015, page 749.

38.

B 12-mm thick/6-mm midline shift

According to current guidelines, any acute subdural hematoma that measures greater than 10 mm in thickness and is associated with greater than 5 mm of midline shift should be surgically evacuated regardless of GCS.

Further Reading: Harbaugh, Shaffrey, Couldwell, Berger. Neurosurgery Knowledge Update, 2015, page 753.

39.

B NSAIDs

There is currently no role for steroids in the treatment of brachial neuritis. These patients are managed conservatively and NSAIDs can be used for shoulder pain.

Further Reading: Harbaugh, Shaffrey, Couldwell, Berger. Neurosurgery Knowledge Update, 2015, page 736.

40.

D 90%

Brachial neuritis is managed conservatively, and most patients experience a full recovery at 3 years. The rate of recovery is around 90%. Supportive care and extensive physical therapy should be utilized in this condition.

Further Reading: Harbaugh, Shaffrey, Couldwell, Berger. Neurosurgery Knowledge Update, 2015, page 736.

41.

C Bradycardia

Precedex is an alpha-2 agonist in the CNS that can be used for sedation. It has dose-dependent effects on blood pressure and heart rate, specifically causing hypotension and bradycardia.

Further Reading: Siddiqi. Neurosurgical Intensive Care, 2017, page 160.

42.

D Locus coeruleus

Precedex is a central alpha-2 agonist that is thought to exert its effects on the locus coeruleus in the brainstem, mediating arousal and sleep–wake cycles. Decreasing transmission of the neurons in this nucleus that are primarily noradrenergic causes sedation and diminishes agitation.

Further Reading: Siddiqi. Neurosurgical Intensive Care, 2017, page 161.

43.

D 24 hours

Currently, the FDA has only approved continuous infusion of Precedex for 24 hours given the risk of rebound hypertension and tachycardia after cessation of administration.

Further Reading: Siddiqi. Neurosurgical Intensive Care, 2017, page 161.

44.

B New right bundle branch block

Propofol infusion syndrome is thought to occur in patients receiving high-dose propofol infusion for more than 48 hours. The exact mechanism is unknown but thought to be due to metabolic derangements in the mitochondria. Initial findings can include a right bundle branch block. It can go on to include hypotension, bradycardia, metabolic acidosis, rhabdomyolysis, and hypokalemia. Propofol should be stopped.

Further Reading: Siddiqi. Neurosurgical Intensive Care, 2017, page 159.

45.

B Etomidate

Etomidate is an anesthetic agent that decreases $CMRO_2$ and cerebral blood flow. It also causes adrenocortical axis suppression and decreases the concentration of ACTH.

Further Reading: Albright, Pollack, Adelson. Principles and Practice of Pediatric Neurosurgery, 3rd edition, 2015, page 740.

46.

A Patent foramen ovale

The sitting position can be useful in neurosurgery, but there is an increased risk of venous air embolism. A patient with a PFO is a relative contraindication for the use of the sitting position due to the risk of a right-sided air embolism becoming a left-sided embolism.

Further Reading: Albright, Pollack, Adelson. Principles and Practice of Pediatric Neurosurgery, 3rd edition, 2015, page 142.

47.

E Methohexital

Methohexital is an anesthetic agent that lowers the seizure threshold. It is sometimes used during electrocorticography for surgical treatment of epilepsy.

Further Reading: Baltuch, Villemure. Operative Techniques in Epilepsy Surgery, 2009, page 48.

48.

D ~ 60%

In patients with refractory temporal lobe epilepsy (TLE), surgical treatment can lead to 60% seizure freedom at 1 year post-op, compared to 8% seizure freedom in patients undergoing medical management alone.

Further Reading: Harbaugh, Shaffrey, Couldwell, Berger. Neurosurgery Knowledge Update, 2015, page 269.

49.

B Temporary motor deficit

Multiple subpial transections can be performed as a palliative epilepsy surgery in patients with medically refractory epilepsy. It severs the horizontal intracortical connections, but preserves neurons due to the vertical columnar orientation. These patients should expect to have transient neurologic deficit for several months postoperatively.

Further Reading: Harbaugh, Shaffrey, Couldwell, Berger. Neurosurgery Knowledge Update, 2015, page 272.

50.

C Temporal lobe

The rising epigastric sensation and déjà vu can be associated with TLE.

Further Reading: Harbaugh, Shaffrey, Couldwell, Berger. Neurosurgery Knowledge Update, 2015, page 264.

51.

D Throbbing pain

Type I, or classic TN, usually presents with sharp, lancinating unilateral pain with pain-free intervals. In studies on the subject, type I patients were more likely to have arterial compression at surgery as well as better long-term outcomes than type II patients, which tend to have persistent, burning/aching/throbbing pain that can be bilateral, and may be associated with other pathologies, such as multiple sclerosis.

Further Reading: Harbaugh, Shaffrey, Couldwell, Berger. Neurosurgery Knowledge Update, 2015, page 294.

52.

D 85%

According to current literature, up to 84% of patients with type I TN pain will experience excellent to good pain control with microvascular decompression surgery.

Further Reading: Harbaugh, Shaffrey, Couldwell, Berger. Neurosurgery Knowledge Update, 2015, page 294.

53.

B 65%

Patients with atypical type II TN may still benefit from microvascular decompression. Up to 65% of these patients will have "excellent to good" pain control long term.

Further Reading: Harbaugh, Shaffrey, Couldwell, Berger. Neurosurgery Knowledge Update, 2015, page 294.

54.

D Medical management

This patient has TN and has not yet undergone any treatment. Initial management should be with carbamazepine, as 80% of patients will experience nearly immediate relief (within 24–48 hours) with this medication. The pain relief diminishes over time, and over the long term, only 50% of patients may have continued relief on carbamazepine. Up to 10% of patients may not tolerate carbamazepine.

Further Reading: Harbaugh, Shaffrey, Couldwell, Berger. Neurosurgery Knowledge Update, 2015, page 295.

55.

A Voltage-gated sodium channel blockade

Oxcarbazepine is a sodium channel blocking pain medication that works in a similar fashion to carbamazepine. It can be used in some patients that cannot tolerate standard carbamazepine.

Further Reading: Harbaugh, Shaffrey, Couldwell, Berger. Neurosurgery Knowledge Update, 2015, page 295.

56.

C Lateral

The distribution of the V1, V2, and V3 divisions of the trigeminal nerve is oriented in the foramen ovale in a superomedial to inferolateral direction. Therefore, to best treat V3 pain, the catheter should be placed lateral within the foramen.

Further Reading: Harbaugh, Shaffrey, Couldwell, Berger. Neurosurgery Knowledge Update, 2015, page 297.

57.

B A 55-year-old male alcoholic

This image demonstrates central pontine my-elinolysis (CPM), also known as osmotic demy-elination syndrome. Patients with alcoholism can experience severe alterations in electrolytes, which could lead to CPM.

Further Reading: Rohkamm. Color Atlas of Neurol-ogy, 2007, page 310.

58.

B Hyperkalemia

Hyperkalemia can cause tall, peaked or spiked T waves on ECG

Further Reading: Citow, Macdonald, Refai. Compre-hensive Neurosurgery Board Review, 2nd edition, 2010, page 519.

59.

B Hypocalcemia

Hypocalcemia can be associated with lengthen-ing of the PR interval on ECG.

Further Reading: Citow, Macdonald, Refai. Compre-hensive Neurosurgery Board Review, 2nd edition, 2010, page 520.

60.

C Multifocality

Hypomagnesemia can cause multifocality on ECG.

Further Reading: Citow, Macdonald, Refai. Compre-hensive Neurosurgery Board Review, 2nd edition, 2010, page 520.

61.

A Cortical-based tumor

The presence of an intracranial tumor, aneu-rysm or arteriovenous malformation (AVM) is absolute contraindication to the administration of IV rtPA for acute ischemic stroke.

Further Reading: Harbaugh, Shaffrey, Couldwell, Berger. Neurosurgery Knowledge Update, 2015, page 10.

62.

B Choroidal point

PICA originates from the vertebral artery and supplies the brainstem and cerebellum. After the choroidal point, PICA is supplying only cerebellum and if needed could be taken with minimal side effects. Proximal to this point, a medullary infarct will likely occur.

Further Reading: Harbaugh, Shaffrey, Couldwell, Berger. Neurosurgery Knowledge Update, 2015, page 16.

63.

A Superior thyroid

The superior thyroid artery is the first branch of the external carotid artery. It is commonly seen and needs to be controlled during carotid endarterectomy.

Further Reading: Harbaugh, Shaffrey, Couldwell, Berger. Neurosurgery Knowledge Update, 2015, page 32.

64.

D Sphenopalatine

The sphenopalatine artery is the primary vas-cular supply to the nasal cavity.

Further Reading: Harbaugh, Shaffrey, Couldwell, Berger. Neurosurgery Knowledge Update, 2015, page 35.

65.

A 4%

Patients with aneurysmal subarachnoid hem-orrhage (SAH) with an unsecured aneurysm are at risk of rebleed, which can have devastating conse-quences. The risk in the first 24 hours is roughly 4%.

Further Reading: Harbaugh, Shaffrey, Couldwell, Berger. Neurosurgery Knowledge Update, 2015, page 45.

66.

B 15 to 20%

There is an elevated risk of aneurysm rebleed in the first 2 weeks after rupture if the aneurysm remains unsecured. That risk is approximately 15 to 20%. The mortality of aneurysm rebleed is near 75%.

Further Reading: Harbaugh, Shaffrey, Couldwell, Berger. Neurosurgery Knowledge Update, 2015, page 45.

67.

B Catecholamine surge

Neurogenic pulmonary edema can occur after aneurysmal SAH and close pulmonary monitoring should occur in these patients. While pulmonary edema can occur from iatrogenic fluid overload, neurogenic pulmonary edema is thought to be due to an acute catecholamine surge experienced after the bleeding event.

Further Reading: Harbaugh, Shaffrey, Couldwell, Berger. Neurosurgery Knowledge Update, 2015, page 46.

68.

A Hyponatremia

The most common electrolyte disturbance in SAH is hyponatremia, which can occur via two mechanisms, either cerebral salt wasting (CSW) or SIADH. It is important to determine volume status to differentiate between SIADH and CSW.

Further Reading: Harbaugh, Shaffrey, Couldwell, Berger. Neurosurgery Knowledge Update, 2015, page 47.

69.

C Anterior communicating artery

Occasionally patients with SAH can present with hypernatremia, caused by diabetes insipidus. This may be suggestive of an anterior communicating artery aneurysm due to destruction of hypothalamic pathways involved in the production and release of ADH.

Further Reading: Harbaugh, Shaffrey, Couldwell, Berger. Neurosurgery Knowledge Update, 2015, page 47.

70.

D Early enteral nutrition

Intubated SAH patients have high rates of gastrointestinal (GI) stress ulcer formation and should all be placed on GI prophylactic medications. Early enteral nutrition via either percutaneous gastrostomy or nasogastric tube can allow for early feeding, thus decreasing stress ulcer formation.

Further Reading: Harbaugh, Shaffrey, Couldwell, Berger. Neurosurgery Knowledge Update, 2015, page 47.

71.

D Poor outcome and decreased ICP

The DECRA trial was performed in Australia in 2011 and demonstrated that patients who underwent decompressive craniectomy (DC) had improvement in their ICP and shorter intensive care unit (ICU) stays, but overall had poorer outcomes than standard care. The trial has been criticized for having too aggressive a surgical arm with refractory ICP defined as 20 mm Hg for more than 15 minutes. This may have led to more patients being operated than necessary. The Randomised Evaluation of Surgery with Craniectomy for Uncontrollable Elevation of Intracranial Pressure (RESCUEicp) trial is ongoing and has increased the time frame required to determine refractory ICP elevation.

Further Reading: Harbaugh, Shaffrey, Couldwell, Berger. Neurosurgery Knowledge Update, 2015, page 776.

72.

B Decreased hematoma volume; no clinical effect

The INTERACT trial aimed to determine if intensive blood pressure control had significant effects on clinical outcome. Intensive blood pressure control (systolic blood pressure [SBP] < 140) decreased overall hematoma size, but it did not have any effect on clinical course. INTERACT 2 is ongoing.

Further Reading: Harbaugh, Shaffrey, Couldwell, Berger. Neurosurgery Knowledge Update, 2015, page 229.

73.

B 5 times

According to current literature, baseline hypertension with SBP > 160 leads to a 5.5 times higher risk of spontaneous ICH compared to patients with good blood pressure control.

Further Reading: Harbaugh, Shaffrey, Couldwell, Berger. Neurosurgery Knowledge Update, 2015, page 231.

74.

B 20%

ICH can be a devastating event, and many patients develop neurologic deficits following this event. The rate of functional independence 3 months after the bleeding event occurs is roughly 20%.

Further Reading: Harbaugh, Shaffrey, Couldwell, Berger. Neurosurgery Knowledge Update, 2015, page 231.

75.

E 100%

This patient has suffered a devastating cerebellar hemorrhage that will have a 100% 30-day mortality according to the ICH score. Points are awarded for age older than 80 years, infratentorial location, IVH, hematoma volume greater than 30 mL, and 1 point for GCS 5 to 12. This gives her 5 of a total of 6 points. Patients with an ICH score of

5 or 6 have a 100% 30-day mortality. Patients with a score of 4 have a 97% 30-day mortality.

Further Reading: Harbaugh, Shaffrey, Couldwell, Berger. Neurosurgery Knowledge Update, 2015, page 231.

76.

C Superficial cortical (< 1 cm from the surface) location

In the initial STICH trial, there was no benefit from surgical resection of spontaneous cerebral hemorrhage when compared to standard medical therapy. Upon subgroup analysis, there may be a benefit to resecting a cerebral hemorrhage with a superficial location and significant mass effect. STICH II examined cases of lobar hemorrhage, however, and found no improvement in outcome between the surgical and medical arms of treatment.

Further Reading: Harbaugh, Shaffrey, Couldwell, Berger. Neurosurgery Knowledge Update, 2015, page 232.

77.

A Hypertension

This CT scan demonstrates a cerebellar hemorrhage with intraventricular extension. The most common underlying cause for this disorder is uncontrolled hypertension.

Further Reading: Harbaugh, Shaffrey, Couldwell, Berger. Neurosurgery Knowledge Update, 2015, page 235.

78.

C 50%

This patient has a spontaneous cerebellar hemorrhage and the data suggest that there is a 50% chance of good outcome (Glasgow Outcome Score 4 or 5, meaning no requirement for assistance in activities of daily living) in patients treated surgically for this condition.

Further Reading: Harbaugh, Shaffrey, Couldwell, Berger. Neurosurgery Knowledge Update, 2015, page 236.

79.

D Hydrocephalus

According to American Heart Association (AHA)/American Stroke Association (ASA) ICH guidelines, the presence of neurological deterioration, brainstem compression and/or the presence

of hydrocephalus should make you strongly consider surgical resection of the hematoma and decompression of the posterior fossa. CSF diversion should also be utilized during the surgery. EVD placement alone without hematoma resection is not recommended.

Further Reading: Harbaugh, Shaffrey, Couldwell, Berger. Neurosurgery Knowledge Update, 2015, page 237.

80.

C 3 cm

Three centimeters has been identified as a rough cutoff whereby patients with a hematoma smaller than 3 cm in dimension are less likely to deteriorate and require surgical intervention compared to patients with a hematoma greater than 3 cm. This is not a hard and fast rule, however, and many other factors, including location, brainstem compression, medical comorbidities, and other systemic characteristics, play into the surgical AU2 n making from patient to patient.

Further Reading: Harbaugh, Shaffrey, Couldwell, Berger. Neurosurgery Knowledge Update, 2015, page 237.

81.

C Vasculitis

This pathologic specimen demonstrates arterial wall necrosis and monocytic infiltration of the vessel walls. There is associated granuloma formation. These findings are consistent with vasculitis. Conventional angiogram may demonstrate arterial nicking.

Further Reading: Harbaugh, Shaffrey, Couldwell, Berger. Neurosurgery Knowledge Update, 2015, page 253.

82.

E Decreased ventricular compliance

NPH is characterized by ambulatory difficulties, cognitive impairment, and urinary incontinence in patients with ventriculomegaly but normal CSF pressure. The full underlying mechanism is not well understood, but thought to be due to poor craniospinal compliance of the ventricular system, at least in part.

Further Reading: Harbaugh, Shaffrey, Couldwell, Berger. Neurosurgery Knowledge Update, 2015, page 324.

83.

D Improved gait after high-volume LP

In patients with suspected NPH, high-volume lumbar puncture (LP) should be performed (30–50 mL removed), and gait analysis should be performed immediately after this procedure. Patients who had gait improvement after LP had the highest rate of overall symptom improvement after permanent VP shunt placement.

Further Reading: Harbaugh, Shaffrey, Couldwell, Berger. Neurosurgery Knowledge Update, 2015, page 326.

84.

D Arachnoid cyst

This patient has an arachnoid cyst of the right sylvian fissure. The cyst contents have the same signal intensity as CSF and this is helpful for the diagnosis.

Further Reading: Harbaugh, Shaffrey, Couldwell, Berger. Neurosurgery Knowledge Update, 2015, page 349.

85.

E No improvement in ICP, no clinical improvement, increased systemic complications

Similar to adult TBI, there is no role for systemic steroids in pediatric patients that have severe TBI. Clinical and ICP outcomes show no difference and patients are exposed to systemic risk with steroid administration.

Further Reading: Harbaugh, Shaffrey, Couldwell, Berger. Neurosurgery Knowledge Update, 2015, page 398.

86.

B 24 to 26 weeks of gestation

Currently, fetal surgery for the repair of myelomeningocele occurs at 24 to 26 weeks of gestation.

Further Reading: Harbaugh, Shaffrey, Couldwell, Berger. Neurosurgery Knowledge Update, 2015, page 403.

87.

D Further imaging

This is a young patient with no significant risk factors for spontaneous ICH. The age, lack of risk factors, and odd location of this hemorrhage should make you concerned for an underlying vascular malformation or aneurysm. A CT angiogram (CTA) should be obtained as a start, and likely a formal catheter angiogram to follow depending on the CTA findings.

Further Reading: Harbaugh, Shaffrey, Couldwell, Berger. Neurosurgery Knowledge Update, 2015, page 422.

88.

C Hereditary hemorrhagic telangiectasia

The catheter angiogram demonstrates a cerebral AVM. Of the listed choices, HHT is associated with AVM formation.

Further Reading: Harbaugh, Shaffrey, Couldwell, Berger. Neurosurgery Knowledge Update, 2015, page 424.

89.

A < 10%

With successful indirect or direct bypass in patients with moyamoya disease, the 5-year rate of stroke drops from 67 to 90% to less than 10%.

Further Reading: Harbaugh, Shaffrey, Couldwell, Berger. Neurosurgery Knowledge Update, 2015, page 424.

90.

B Optic chiasm involvement

Optic gliomas in patients with NF1 can be surgically resected en bloc (or nearly en bloc) if it is obvious that there is normal optic nerve on either side of the involved area. In these cases, the tumor can be resected with the optic nerve (and orbit); however, if there is tumor invasion into the optic chiasm, the mass cannot be completely excised without unacceptable risk of bilateral blindness postop.

Further Reading: Harbaugh, Shaffrey, Couldwell, Berger. Neurosurgery Knowledge Update, 2015, page 429.

91.

A Moment arm

Spine biomechanics can be helpful to understand when evaluating traumatic injury to the spine. Forces are applied to the spine in force vectors. When one of these vectors is applied at a given distance from an axis of rotation, a moment arm is created. This moment arm depicts a lever that starts from the IAR to the force application. This property helps explain compression fractures versus burst fracture pathology.

Further Reading: Harbaugh, Shaffrey, Couldwell, Berger. Neurosurgery Knowledge Update, 2015, page 451.

92.

B Force applied per unit area

Stress is defined as force applied per unit area. Strain is defined as change in unit length compared to original length.

Further Reading: Harbaugh, Shaffrey, Couldwell, Berger. Neurosurgery Knowledge Update, 2015, page 452.

93.

B The slope of the most linear region of the force deformation curve

Stiffness of the implant is defined as the slope of the line on the force deformation curve.

Further Reading: Harbaugh, Shaffrey, Couldwell, Berger. Neurosurgery Knowledge Update, 2015, page 453.

94.

C Yield point

The point on the force deformation curve where the implant begins to deform but has not yet undergone complete failure is called the elastic zone. The point where the device enters the elastic zone is termed the yield point.

Further Reading: Harbaugh, Shaffrey, Couldwell, Berger. Neurosurgery Knowledge Update, 2015, page 454.

95.

E 95%

Development of spondylosis in the spine is a normal aspect of aging, and approximately 10% of patients aged 25 years will have spondylosis on imaging, with this percentage increasing to 95% by 65 years of age.

Further Reading: Harbaugh, Shaffrey, Couldwell, Berger. Neurosurgery Knowledge Update, 2015, page 458.

96.

C Excitation of recurrent sinuvertebral nerve endings

Discogenic axial back pain is a controversial issue, especially regarding treatment options, but is thought to occur due to excitation of the

sinuvertebral nerve (a branch from the anterior ramus) that innervates the posterior longitudinal ligament (PLL) and annulus. In patients with spondylosis, irritation, and inflammation of the various structures of the ventral canal are thought to excite these fibers and generate pain.

Further Reading: Harbaugh, Shaffrey, Couldwell, Berger. Neurosurgery Knowledge Update, 2015, page 458.

97.

C Posterior spinal nerve ramus

Facetogenic axial back pain is controversial, but pain from the facet joints is thought to arise from innervating fibers from the posterior ramus of the associated spinal nerve.

Further Reading: Harbaugh, Shaffrey, Couldwell, Berger. Neurosurgery Knowledge Update, 2015, page 458.

98.

C 1,200-mg calcium, 1,000-IU vitamin D

According to NOF guidelines, women older than 50 years should receive 1,200 mg of calcium on a daily basis as well as 1,000 IU of vitamin D.

Further Reading: Harbaugh, Shaffrey, Couldwell, Berger. Neurosurgery Knowledge Update, 2015, page 487.

99.

B Inhibits osteoclasts

Calcitonin antagonizes parathyroid hormone and therefore inhibits osteoclast activity. This decreases bone resorption and helps strengthen bones.

Further Reading: Harbaugh, Shaffrey, Couldwell, Berger. Neurosurgery Knowledge Update, 2015, page 487.

100.

C Increased risk of DVT

Raloxifene is a selective estrogen receptor modifier that is used for bone health. It simultaneously decreases risk of breast cancer and inhibits bone resorption. Patients should be aware of the increased risk of DVT with the administration of raloxifene.

Further Reading: Harbaugh, Shaffrey, Couldwell, Berger. Neurosurgery Knowledge Update, 2015, page 487.